MCQs for GPVTS

CLINICAL SPECIALTIES

David R Phillips MA MBBChir MRCP DipGUM

Edited by Ruth V Reed MA MBBChir MRCPCH

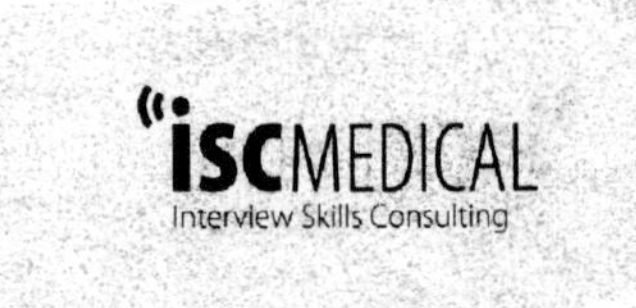

Published by ISCMedical
Suite 434, Hamilton House, Mabledon Place, London WC1H 9BB
Tel: 0845 226 9487

First Published: January 2006
Second Edition: May 2006

ISBN13: 978-1-905812-02-8
ISBN10: 1-905812-02-7
A catalogue record for this book is available from the British Library.

The author has, as far as possible, taken care to ensure that the information given in this text is accurate and up to date. However, readers are strongly advised to confirm that the information with regards to specific patient management complies with current legislation, guidelines and local protocols.

The information within this text is intended as a study aid for the purpose of the GPVTS selection examinations. It is not intended, nor should it be used as a medical reference for the direct management of patients or their conditions.

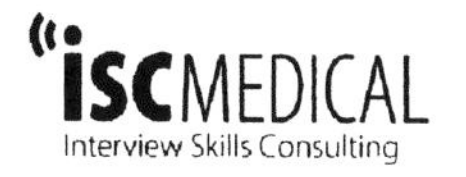

To Paula & Martyn

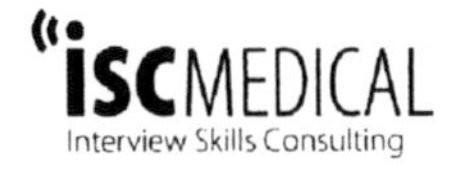

PREFACE

Over the last decade, applications for GPVTS have become more and more competitive. To help select the best applicants, formal assessment with MCQs (Multiple Choice Questions) or EMQs (Extended Matching Questions) alongside interviews are now obligatory for many deaneries. This book aims to give you practice in the types of MCQs you may be faced with.

Candidates are not expected to have highly specialist knowledge. This is an entrance exam into a general training program after all. What is expected is a knowledge base founded from good undergraduate education that has developed with professional experience. In other words, what one would expect of any competent, sensible "House/pre-registration Doctor". For this purpose, the questions attempt to determine whether candidates have indeed taken an active role in their jobs and testing whether candidates are able to demonstrate logical thinking and common sense.

Before you dive into the questions, take a moment to read the following advice. Firstly, I know you have heard it before but, **if** there is **no** negative marking then answer EVERY question. Some people still leave questions blank! Next, think about the phraseology of the questions. See below:

Term	**Meaning**
Pathognomic	A feature which when present is diagnostic for a condition. E.g. Koplik spots in measles.
Characteristic (or typical)	A feature which, if present, highly suggests the diagnosis and if absent would lead you to question the diagnosis. Example: Chest pain and myocardial infarction.
Common (or mostly)	A feature that occurs more than 50% of the time. E.g. Productive cough with pneumonia.
Recognised (or associated)	An accepted feature of that disease even if it doesn't occur in every case. E.g. Erythema nodosum and Crohn's colitis

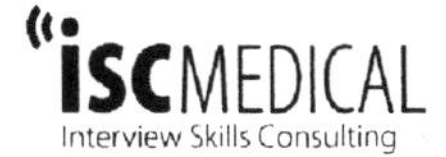

Rare — A feature or condition which one would expect with a low frequency i.e. <1-2%

Specificity — The ability of a test or criteria to pick up a case whilst excluding negatives i.e. few false positives. See below

Specific — A test or criteria which if positive will identify a disease or organism, but no other i.e. few false positives. E.g. Troponin I for myocardial injury.

Sensitivity — The ability of a test or criteria to pick up as many cases as possible without missing any i.e. few false negatives. See below.

Sensitive — A test or criteria that is able to identify cases of a disease. E.g. Amylase in diagnosing pancreatitis.

Understanding the grammar also helps. There was a rhyme at medical school that went: “Never say never nor ever say always”. This refers to the fact that, features in medicine rarely occur all of the time or none of the time. With this in mind, statements such as; “Disease X always presents with Y.” or “Patients with condition A never have feature B.” tend to be false. So if in doubt with such a question, ticking ‘false’ is a useful strategy. The opposite tends to occur for the words ‘may be’ or ‘can be’. They allow for the possibility that rare exceptions to the rules creep in. Such statements then tend to be true. For example “Cystic fibrosis treatment may involve liver transplantation.” This is certainly not the case for every patient but rarely happens and so is true. Since many candidates now catch on to these tricks, examiners try to avoid these terms. However be warned! There are cases when by definition the response MUST be true. For example “Cushing’s disease is always caused by an increased secretion of ACTH from the pituitary gland.” It must be true since the statement is the definition of Cushing’s disease.

Keep these tips in mind and have plenty of practice. That and a good night’s sleep before the exam will keep your wits about you. And don’t forget to READ THE QUESTION CAREFULLY!

Best of Luck
D.R.P

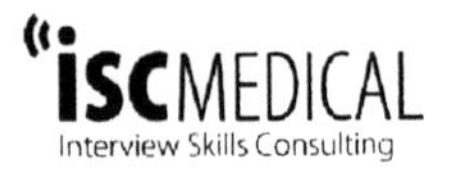

GLOSSARY

ACE	Angiotensin converting enzyme
AIDS	Acquired immunodeficiency syndrome
ALT	Alanine transferase
APTT	Activated partial thromboplastin time
ASD	Atrial septal defect
BCG	Bacille Calmette-Guérin
CEA	Carcinoembryonic antigen
CPK	Creatanine phosphokinase
CRP	C reactive protein
CT	Computed tomography
CVA	Cerebrovascular accident
DIC	Disseminated intravascular coagulation
DVT	Deep vein thrombosis
ECG	Electrocardiogram
EEG	Electroencephalography
ESR	Erythrocyte sedimentation rate
GTN	Glyceryl trinitrate
HCG	Human chorionic gonadotrophin
HHV8	Human herpes virus 8
HIV	Human immunodeficiency virus
INR	International normalised ratio
IUCD	Intrautarine contraceptive device
IUD	Intrauterine(contraceptive) device

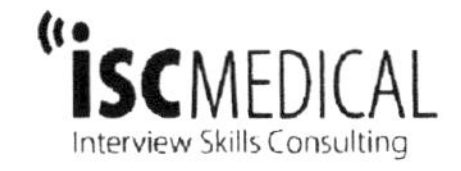

JVP	Jugular venous pressure
LDH	Lactate dehydrogenase
MRI	Magnetic resonance imaging
NICE	National institute for clinical excellence
NSAID	Non-steroidal anti-inflammatory drug
PA	Posterior-anterior
PCR	Polymerase chain reaction
PDA	Patent ductus arteriosus
PET	Positron emission tomography
PT	Prothrombin time
RAST	Radioallergosorbent test
SIADH	Syndrome of inappropriate antidiuretic hormone secretion
SLE	Systemic lupus erythromatosis
TB	Tuberculosis
TIA	Transient ischaemic attack
TNF	Tumour necrosis factor
TSH	Thyroid stimulating hormone
UV	Ultra-Violet
VDRL	Venereal disease research laboratory
VSD	Ventricular septal defect
WCC	White cell count

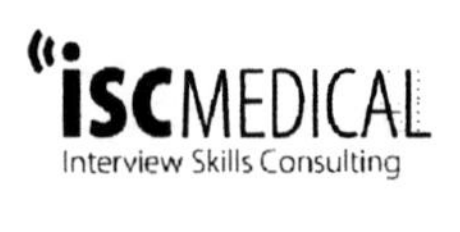
iSCMEDICAL
Interview Skills Consulting

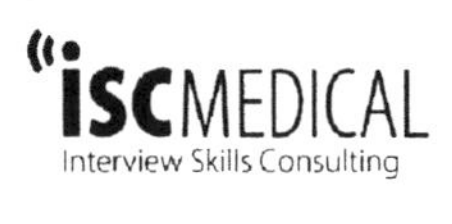

CONTENTS

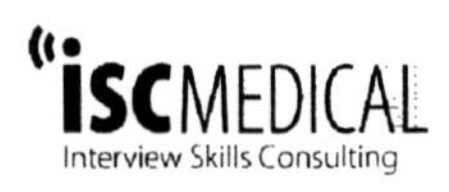
iSCMEDICAL
Interview Skills Consulting

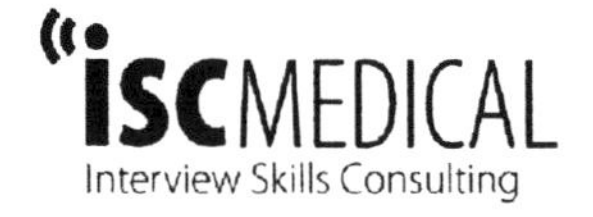

MCQs for GPVTS

DERMATOLOGY

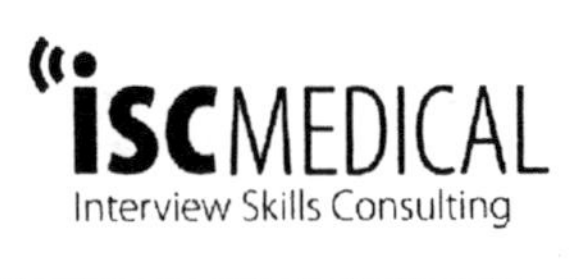

1 The following are common indications for the use of lasers. **DERM**

a. Port wine stains. True/False

b. Pigmented naevi. True/False

c. Keloid scars. True/False

d. Tattoo removal. True/False

e. Strawberry naevi. True/False

2 Atopic eczema in a child. **DERM**

a. Is complicated by superficial skin infections and bleeding from excoriations. True/False

b. Elimination diets are often able to identify a trigger which, once excluded, reduces further disease burden. True/False

c. The risk can be reduced if soya milk is given during infancy. True/False

d. Allowing a child to scratch only at certain times of the week or day is a useful strategy to help break the scratch itch cycle. True/False

e. Absence of scratch or itch makes the diagnosis very unlikely. True/False

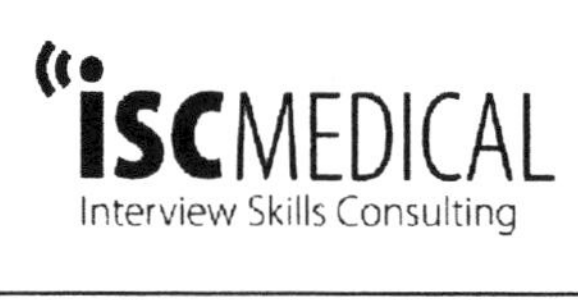

3	Infection may have a significant role in the following skin conditions.	DERM

a. Seborrhoeic dermatitis. True/False

b. Acne rosacea. True/False

c. Molluscum contagiosum. True/False

d. Pityriasis versicolor. True/False

e. Keloid. True/False

4	Bacterial skin infections.	DERM

a. Erysipelas is a superficial skin infection, yet causes fever and raised white cell count. True/False

b. Erysipelas is most often attributed to staphylococcal infection. True/False

c. Erysipelas is characterised by golden crusted lesions on an erythematous base. True/False

d. Impetigo is a superficial skin infection in which topical fusidic acid or oral antibiotics are adequate treatments. True/False

e. Impetigo has a predilection for flexures and skin creases. True/False

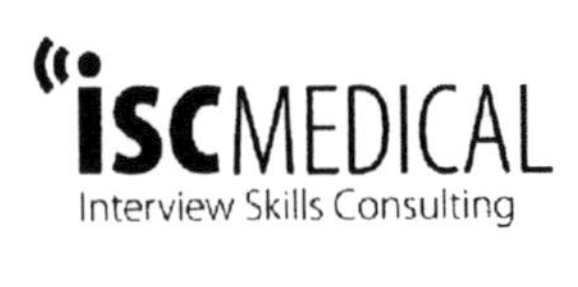

5	Acne vulgaris.	DERM

a. The comedone is white (white head) when full of pus and black if mild haemorrhage has occurred. True/False

b. Is worsened by 'junk food' diet. True/False

c. Pathogenesis is secondary to sweat gland hypersensivity to androgens and subsequent blocking. True/False

d. Emollients are useful when acne remedies dry the skin. True/False

e. The presence of any lesions other than on the face signifies moderate or severe disease. True/False

6	Management of acne vulgaris.	DERM

a. Often an oral and topical antibiotic is used. If so they should be different types as a 'combination' therapy. True/False

b. Oral antibiotics are rarely used for mild acne. True/False

c. Short courses of oral antibiotic therapy are useful adjuncts to management. True/False

d. Retinoic acid compounds are reserved for severe forms or those with significant psychological distress. True/False

e. Individuals have an increased risk of developing acne rosacea in later life. True/False

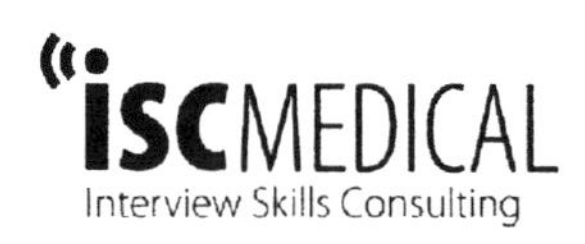

7 Acne rosacea. **DERM**

a. Is associated with alcohol intake. True/False

b. Is characterised by pustules, comedones and telangectasia. True/False

c. Conjunctivitis is a recognised complication. True/False

d. Keratitis is a recognised complication. True/False

e. Uveitis is a recognised complication. True/False

8 The following is true regarding lichen planus. **DERM**

a. It is a associated with HLA-CW6. True/False

b. It is a cause of scarring alopecia. True/False

c. It can cause nail ridging. True/False

d. Wickham's striae are white lacy markings only seen on the surface of mucosal lesions. True/False

e. Local lymph nodes are commonly enlarged. True/False

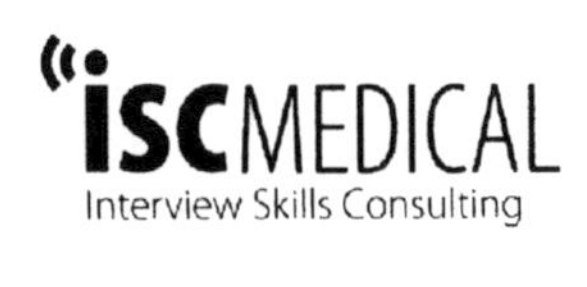

9	The following statements are true.	DERM

a. The herald patch in pityriasis rosea is of the same morphology as later lesions. True/False

b. Human herpes viruses have been implicated in pityriasis rosea. True/False

c. Pemphigoid is characterised by the presence of linear IgA and complement along the basement membrane on biopsy. True/False

d. Pemphigus is characterised by autoantibodies directed against tissue components that stabilise intradermal structures. True/False

e. Oral steroids are preferred to topical treatments in pemphigoid as opposed to pemphigus where topical treatments are favoured. True/False

10	The following skin lesions are correctly paired with a recognised cause.	DERM

a. Erythema marginatum : Rheumatic fever. True/False

b. Erythema multiforme : Mycoplasma pneumonia. True/False

c. Erythema chronicum migrans (ECM) : Leptospirosis. True/False

d. Livedo reticularis : Crohn's colitis. True/False

e. Erythema ab igne : Peripheral neuropathy leading to excessive heat exposure. True/False

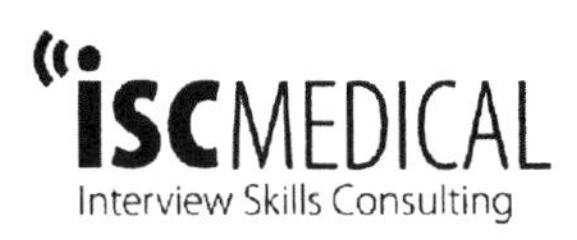

11	The following is true regarding scabies.	DERM

a. Genital lesions tend to be nodular or papular. True/False

b. Itch is worse at night. True/False

c. Symptoms usually appear around 4 weeks after infection. True/False

d. Topical treatments must be left on for 24 hours before washing off. True/False

e. All household members and pets must be treated. True/False

12	The following is true of atopic eczema.	DERM

a. Hydrocortisone is contraindicated on the face because of the risk of later telangectasia. True/False

b. Is associated with an excessive TH1 reaction. True/False

c. Very greasy emollients are the best but are unacceptable to many young patients. True/False

d. Nickel is a common trigger. True/False

e. Staphylococcus aureus in implicated. True/False

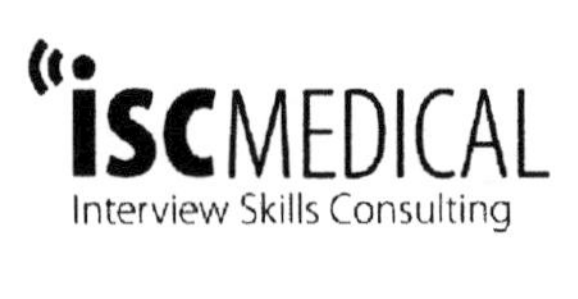

13	The following skin conditions may be related to HIV.	DERM

a. Norwegian scabies. True/False

b. Eosinophilic folliculitis. True/False

c. Pyogenic granulomata. True/False

d. HHV8 associated sarcoma. True/False

e. Lichen planus. True/False

14	The following are recognised dermatological associations with diabetes mellitus.	DERM

a. Intertrigo. True/False

b. Folliculitis. True/False

c. Pyoderma gangrenosum. True/False

d. Granuloma annulare. True/False

e. Necrobiosis lipoidica. True/False

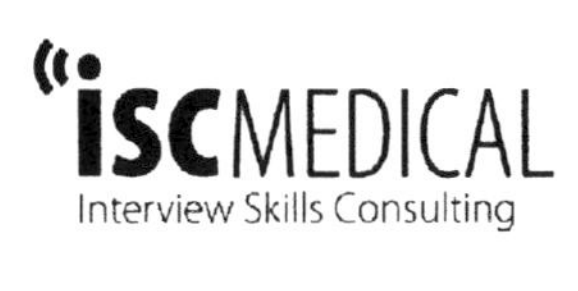

15	The following are conditions which typically give ring shaped skin lesions.	DERM

a. Tinea corporis. True/False

b. Erythema chronicum migrans. True/False

c. Pompholyx eczema. True/False

d. Circinate balanitis. True/False

e. Discoid lupus. True/False

16	Management of advanced psoriasis.	DERM

a. Diprobase is the mainstay background treatment for many patients. True/False

b. Methotrexate is a useful oral treatment. True/False

c. Pregnancy must be avoided for up to 2 years after using Acitretin. True/False

d. Rituximab shows promise for moderate to severe arthritis. True/False

e. UVB therapy is especially useful for guttate psoriasis. True/False

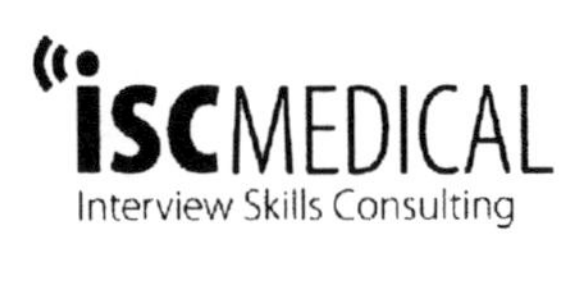

17	The following conditions typically cause itching.	DERM

a. Pityriasis versicolor. True/False

b. Dermatitis herpetiformis. True/False

c. Lichen planus. True/False

d. Chloasma. True/False

e. Lichen sclerosus. True/False

18	The following conditions demonstrate the Köbner phenomenon.	DERM

a. Lichenification. True/False

b. Lichen planus. True/False

c. Vitiligo. True/False

d. Psoriasis. True/False

e. Molluscum contagiosum. True/False

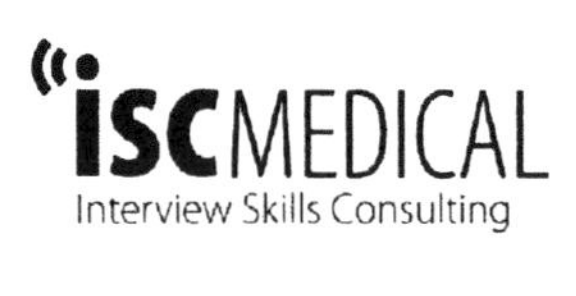

19 The following is associated with underlying gastrointestinal disease. **DERM**

a. Acanthosis nigricans. True/False

b. Erythema nodosum. True/False

c. Eczema herpeticum. True/False

d. Tylosis. True/False

e. Pyoderma gangrenosum. True/False

20 The following are common associations of erythema multiforme. **DERM**

a. Haemophilus influenzae. True/False

b. Amoxicillin. True/False

c. Mycoplasma pneumonia. True/False

d. Sarcoidosis. True/False

e. Lyme disease. True/False

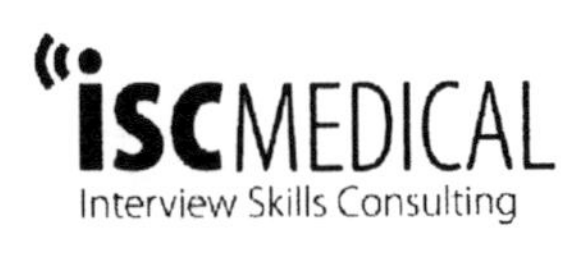

21 The following is true of a basal cell carcinoma. **DERM**

a. Superficial telangectasia is a hallmark feature. True/False

b. Can occur on the chest as a scaly plaque. True/False

c. It virtually never metastasises. True/False

d. Radiotherapy is part of the management plan for some lesions. True/False

e. Has a typical shallow ulcer almost flat with the surrounding skin. True/False

22 The following are recognised risk factors for the development of squamous cell carcinoma of the skin. **DERM**

a. Vitamin C deficiency. True/False

b. Human papilloma virus. True/False

c. Sunlight. True/False

d. Venous leg disease. True/False

e. Smoking. True/False

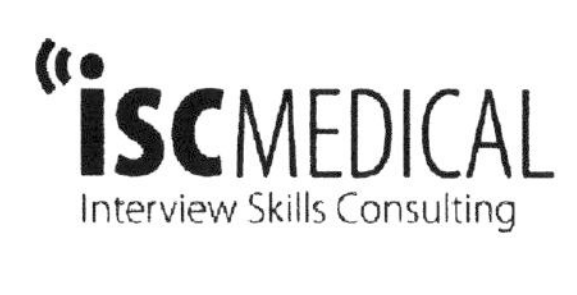

23	Melanoma and sun exposure.	DERM

a. The majority of melanomas arise from pre-existing naevi. True/False

b. A Breslow thickness score of < 1mm confers a 5 year survival rate >90%. True/False

c. Sunscreens protect against UVA and UVB only. True/False

d. The sun screen factor refers to how much longer than normal for them an individual can stay out in the sun before they will tan. True/False

e. The fairest skin types (types 4 and 5) are more prone to melanoma. True/False

24	The following are recognised triggers of psoriasis.	DERM

a. Sunlight. True/False

b. Stopping steroids. True/False

c. Lithium. True/False

d. Beta blockers. True/False

e. Streptococcal infection. True/False

25 The following atypical sites may be involved in psoriasis. **DERM**

a. Inframammary fold. True/False

b. Umbilicus. True/False

c. Axillae. True/False

d. Behind the ear. True/False

e. First interdigital space on the hands. True/False

26 Management of psoriasis. **DERM**

a. Tar based treatments are dangerous if in contact with children. True/False

b. Vitamin D analogues, if applied in large quantities to inflamed skin, may lead to systemic effects such as hypercalcaemia. True/False

c. Tar based treatments are available over the counter and are safe for scalp use. True/False

d. Flexural psoriasis is best treated with steroid type agents. True/False

e. Dithranol is practical as a scalp lotion used as a shampoo. True/False

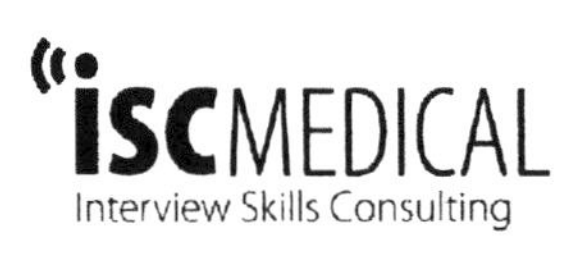

27	The following conditions give rise to well demarcated discrete round or oval lesions.	DERM

a. Pityriasis rosea. True/False

b. Lichen planus. True/False

c. Guttate psoriasis. True/False

d. Ichthyosis. True/False

e. Erythema ab igne. True/False

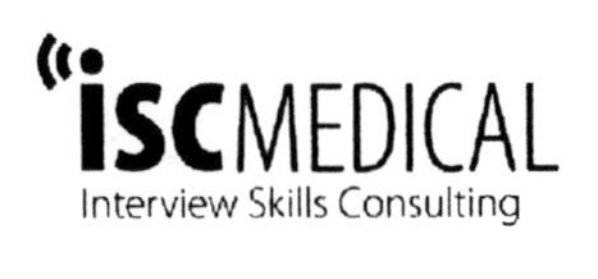
iscMEDICAL
Interview Skills Consulting

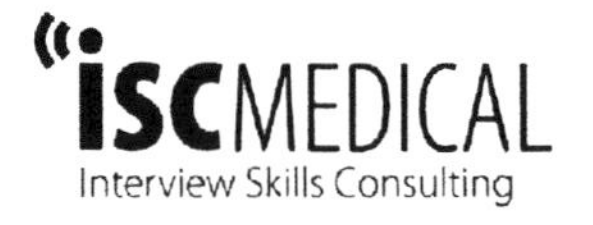

MCQs for GPVTS

ENT

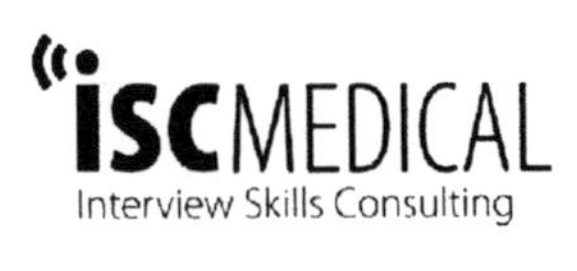

28 Causes of chronic rhinorrhoea include the following. **ENT**

a. NSAIDs. True/False

b. Nasal decongestants. True/False

c. Pregnancy. True/False

d. Asthma. True/False

e. Cystic fibrosis. True/False

29 Allergic rhinitis. **ENT**

a. Certain vasoactive decongestants are contraindicated in ischaemic heart disease. True/False

b. Radio-allergosorbent tests (RAST) look for serum immunoglobulin, which is indicative of delayed type hypersensitivity to a range of common allergens. True/False

c. Sodium cromoglycate spray is contraindicated in asthmatics. True/False

d. Steroid sprays should only be used for up to two weeks at a time otherwise rebound oedema will result leading to return of original symptoms. True/False

e. Desensitisation therapy runs the risk of acute anaphylactic shock. True/False

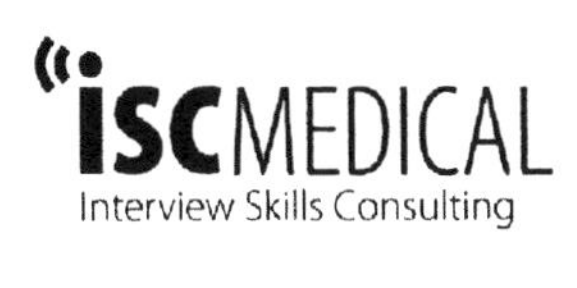

30 Trauma to the nose. **ENT**

a. A 'broken nose' refers to soft tissue injury alone since there is no bone in the nose. True/False

b. A septal haematoma must be referred immediately to an ENT surgeon. True/False

c. In the case of a probable orbital fracture, facial radiographs are not required if a CT scan is performed. True/False

d. Reduction of a 'fracture' can be delayed up to 2 weeks after trauma. True/False

e. Nose blowing is contraindicated post operatively. True/False

31 The following are recognised causes of perforation of the nasal septum. **ENT**

a. Crack cocaine. True/False

b. Basal cell carcinoma. True/False

c. Crohn's disease. True/False

d. Tuberculosis. True/False

e. Herpes zoster virus. True/False

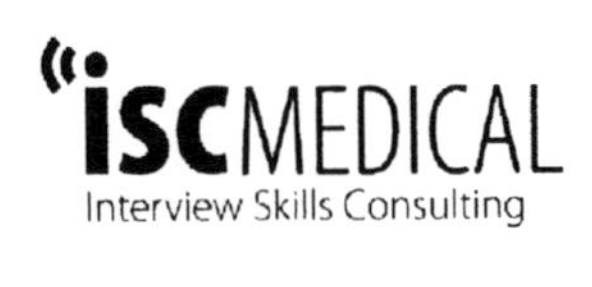

32	The following are recognised causes and associations of epistaxis.	ENT

a. Hypertension. True/False

b. Alcoholism. True/False

c. Nasal oxygen delivery. True/False

d. Cold weather. True/False

e. Foreign body. True/False

33	Nasal polyps.	ENT

a. Are painless. True/False

b. Often give a purulent nasal discharge. True/False

c. Steroid sprays may be suitable treatment. True/False

d. Surgery requires anaesthesia. True/False

e. Orbital involvement can occur. True/False

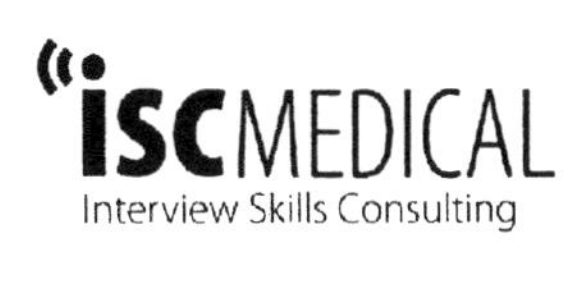

34 The following is true regarding epistaxis. ENT

a. A patient should have his or her head held back to reduce blood trickling forward. True/False

b. In haemodynamically stable patients, initial care involves ice packs and pinching the bridge of the nose. True/False

c. Insertion and inflation of a foley catheter is a recommended method for stabilising posterior bleeds. True/False

d. Packing should only be performed once the site of bleeding is determined. True/False

e. Anterior bleeds tend to be minor compared with posterior bleeds. True/False

35 The following is true regarding sinusitis. ENT

a. Most cases of sinusitis are due to a bacterial infection. True/False

b. Most cases of acute sinusitis should involve management in the community with oral antibiotics. True/False

c. Altered taste sensation is a recognised feature. True/False

d. Cavernous sinus thrombosis is a recognised complication. True/False

e. Swelling is rare and is suggestive of underlying dental problems or carcinoma. True/False

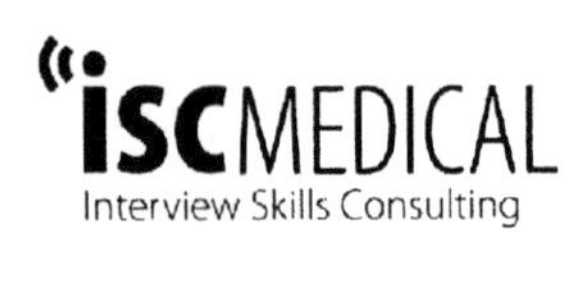

36 The tonsils. **ENT**

a. Squamous cell carcinomas may present with sore throat, dysphonia or ear pain. True/False

b. Haemorrhage a week after tonsillectomy usually requires revision surgery. True/False

c. Amoxicillin is contraindicated in the treatment of tonsillitis. True/False

d. Tonsillitis is often caused by group B streptococcus. True/False

e. An inability to swallow saliva suggests a quinsy during an attack of tonsillitis. True/False

37 The following are indications for tonsillectomy. **ENT**

a. Wegener's granulomatosis. True/False

b. Obstruction leading to obstructive sleep apnoea. True/False

c. Chronic sinusitis. True/False

d. Peritonsillar abscess. True/False

e. More than 3 attacks per year for more than 3 days over a 2 year period. True/False

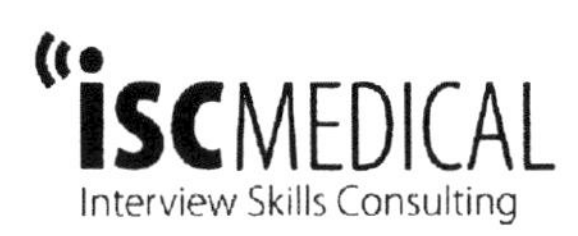

38 The following are recognised causes of chronic laryngitis. **ENT**

a. Rheumatoid arthritis True/False

b. Amateur singing. True/False

c. Wegener's granulomatosis. True/False

d. Mumps. True/False

e. Spicy foods. True/False

39 Benign positional vertigo. **ENT**

a. The condition is often self-limiting within months of presentation. True/False

b. Is a recognised consequence of head injury. True/False

c. Attacks last for only a few seconds at a time. True/False

d. Romberg's test is negative. True/False

e. Laser ablation to posterior semicircular canal is a treatment option. True/False

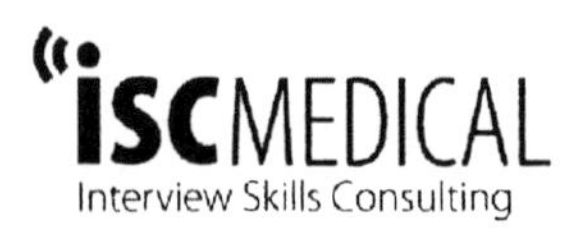

40	Regarding the parotid gland.	ENT

a. Parotid stones are often treated by ultrasonic lithiasis. True/False

b. Parotid stones typically give pain and swelling when drinking sour substances. True/False

c. Mumps parotitis is virtually always bilateral. True/False

d. Any parotid swelling present for more than a month should be referred for further analysis. True/False

e. The majority of tumours of the parotid gland are benign. True/False

41	The following are recognised features and complications of cholesteatoma.	ENT

a. Facial nerve palsy. True/False

b. Vertigo. True/False

c. Headache. True/False

d. Acoustic neuroma. True/False

e. Cerebral abscess. True/False

42	The following are recognised causes of xerostomia.	ENT

a. Nasal obstruction. True/False

b. Sarcoidosis. True/False

c. Beta blockers. True/False

d. Tricyclic antidepressants. True/False

e. Sjögren's syndrome. True/False

43	The following are recognised causes of recurrent laryngeal nerve palsy.	ENT

a. Tuberculous adenitis. True/False

b. Coarctation of the aorta. True/False

c. Hiatus hernia. True/False

d. Oesophageal carcinoma. True/False

e. Parathyroidectomy. True/False

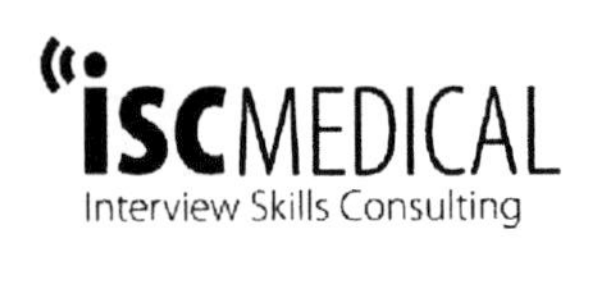

44 The following is true regarding cholesteatoma. **ENT**

a. Is due the invasion of the middle ear by skin tissue. True/False

b. A foul smelling aural discharge is a common complaint. True/False

c. Only occurs as a complication of otitis media. True/False

d. Only occurs as a complication of a perforated ear drum. True/False

e. Wax is broken down to form cholesterol as a by-product of this destructive process. True/False

45 General ear conditions. **ENT**

a. Chondrodermatitis nodularis is an inflammatory reaction thought to be induced by sun and cold exposure. True/False

b. Chondrodermatitis nodularis is often self limiting but, if it persists, topical steroids are effective. True/False

c. Exostoses are benign swellings within the ear canal that may rarely require surgical excision. True/False

d. Wax never originates from the innermost part of the ear canal. True/False

e. Sodium bicarbonate is used to treat ear wax. True/False

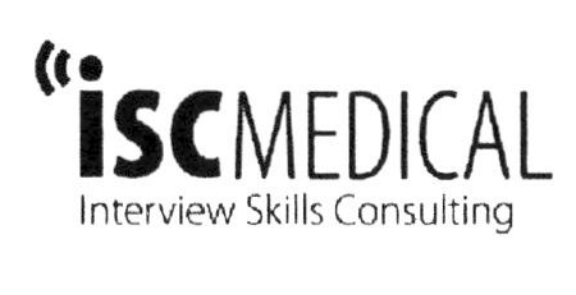

46	The following are acceptable reasons to send a patient to speech therapist.	ENT

a. Anatomical feeding difficulties in an infant. True/False

b. Excessively nasal voice. True/False

c. Unintelligible speech at 3 years of age. True/False

d. Difficulty with sentence structure and word order at 4 years of age. True/False

e. Voice not 'broken' by age 16. True/False

47	Head and neck tumours.	ENT

a. Radiotherapy has a central role in nasopharyngeal carcinoma. True/False

b. Nasopharyngeal carcinoma may present with diplopia or deafness. True/False

c. Iron deficiency anaemia with angular stomatitis are associated with an increased risk of pharyngeal carcinoma. True/False

d. A voice prosthesis is of value in the majority of cases post resection for pharyngeal carcinoma. True/False

e. Hypothyroidism is a late complication following radiotherapy for laryngeal carcinomas. True/False

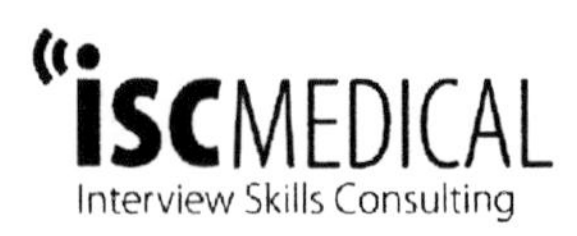

48	Hearing tests.	ENT

a. In conductive deafness, sound localises to the normal ear during the Weber test. True/False

b. Rinne's test is positive in the normal patient. True/False

c. A Barany noise box can be used to prevent the non-tested ear picking up the sound by bone conduction during the Rinne's test. True/False

d. Pure tone audiometry is subjective whereas speech audiometry is an objective measure of hearing. True/False

e. Tympanometry is an objective measure of sensorineural deafness. True/False

49	The following conditions can refer pain to the ear.	ENT

a. Cervical spondylosis. True/False

b. Herpes ophthalmica. True/False

c. Tonsillitis. True/False

d. Dental abscess. True/False

e. Carcinoma of the tongue. True/False

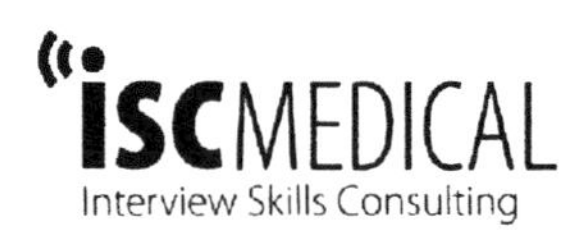

50 'Glue ear'. **ENT**

a. This is the most common cause of hearing impairment in school aged children. True/False

b. Grommets aid hearing by allowing drainage of the middle ear. True/False

c. Swimming is contraindicated while grommets are in place. True/False

d. Eustachian tube dysfunction forms part of the underlying pathophysiology. True/False

e. Cystic fibrosis is a recognised risk factor. True/False

51 Bullous myringitis. **ENT**

a. Is characterised by painful blisters on the ear drum. True/False

b. Pseudomonal species are often implicated. True/False

c. Often leads to a reactive middle ear effusion. True/False

d. Antibiotics are required in only a minority of cases. True/False

e. Steroid based ear drops have a role in persistent inflammation. True/False

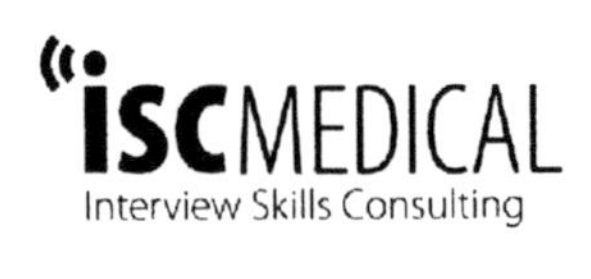

52 Vertigo. ENT

a. Antiemetics are of use in treating acute symptoms of Ménière's disease. True/False

b. Patients will often describe feeling light in the head, as if they have to lie down. True/False

c. Presence of nystagmus indicates a central cause of the vertigo. True/False

d. Vestibular neuronitis is a self limiting condition. True/False

e. Up to 10% of those with vestibular neuronitis may go on to develop Ménière's disease. True/False

53 Discharge from the ear. ENT

a. Fungal infections often give a crumbly discharge with a cheese-like odour. True/False

b. The halo sign on filter paper signifies a potential risk of meningitis. True/False

c. Watery discharge is suggestive of a mainly external ear problem. True/False

d. Blood in the discharge is highly suggestive of ear drum perforation and middle ear involvement. True/False

e. Chronic suppurative otitis media typically gives a painless discharge. True/False

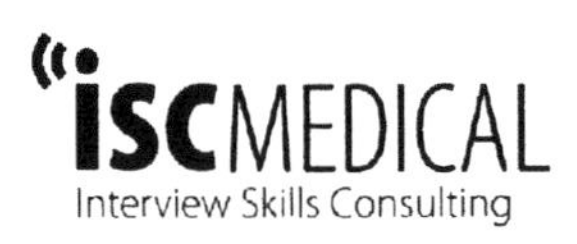

54 The following are recognised features of 'glue ear'. **ENT**

a. Bulging ear drum. True/False

b. Retracted ear drum. True/False

c. Dull ear drum. True/False

d. Yellow ear drum. True/False

e. Superficial vessels seen on ear drum. True/False

55 Otosclerosis. **ENT**

a. Is an autosomal dominant condition. True/False

b. Is a contraindication to the oral contraceptive pill. True/False

c. Surgery involves a stapes implant. True/False

d. Hearing loss is conductive. True/False

e. Tinnitus is a recognised feature. True/False

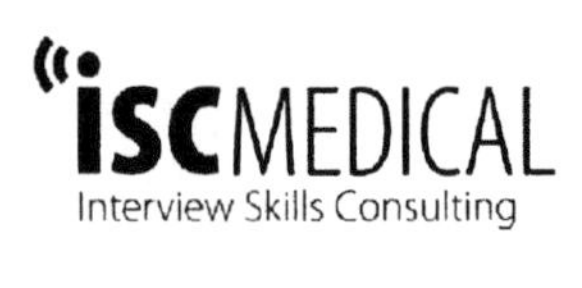

56	Presbyacusis.	ENT

a. Onset is gradual and often before the age of 30. True/False

b. Is more common in those working outdoors. True/False

c. Is more common in those exposed to loud noises (gun blasts). True/False

d. Tends to affect low frequencies first. True/False

e. The presence of background noise makes hearing difficulty worse. True/False

57	The following drugs are associated with the development of tinnitus.	ENT

a. Methylprednisolone. True/False

b. Gentamicin. True/False

c. Aspirin. True/False

d. Spironolactone. True/False

e. Bendrofluazide. True/False

58 Management of tinnitus. **ENT**

a. Hearing aids during the daytime to enhance background noise are beneficial. True/False

b. Benzodiazepines have a reliable role in reducing symptoms and any secondary affective disorder. True/False

c. Cognitive therapy has a role. True/False

d. Ear plugs to block out background noise help with insomnia. True/False

e. If severe, anticonvulsants are useful to reduce neural stimulation. True/False

59 Infections of the outer ear. **ENT**

a. Furunculosis refers to an infection of a hair follicle, usually staphylococcal in origin. True/False

b. If severe or poorly treated, a furunculosis often leads to a discharging otitis externa. True/False

c. Skull infection and meningitis are recognised complications of otitis externa. True/False

d. Antibiotics such as flucloxacillin or penicillin are the best choice for most otitis externa. True/False

e. Prolonged use of aural antibiotics runs the risk of developing fungal infections. True/False

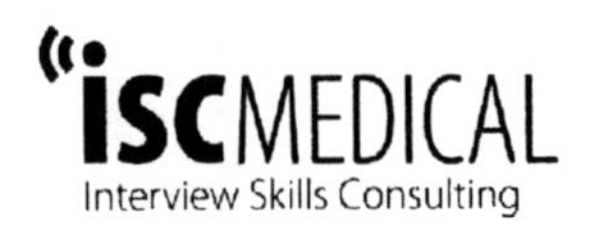
iscMEDICAL
Interview Skills Consulting

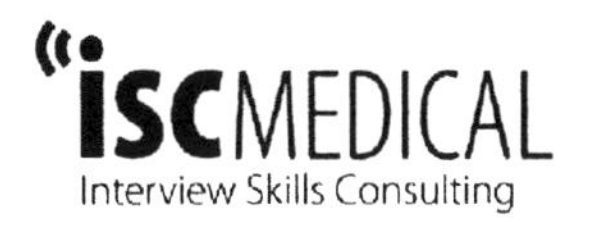

MCQs for GPVTS

GYNAECOLOGY

60 Tests in subfertility. GYNAE

a. Hysterosalpingiogram may require sedation. True/False

b. Post coital cervical mucus can be tested for the presence of sperm. True/False

c. Hysterosalpingiogram is invasive and the procedure should include provision of prophylactic antibiotics. True/False

d. A colposcopy is of use to indicate cervical os anomalies or cervicitis. True/False

e. Thyroid functions are an essential component of the female's hormone profile. True/False

61 Bartholin's glands. GYNAE

a. They are an embryological remnant that persist in up 20% of women. True/False

b. They can lead to cyst formation particularly in those using deodorants. True/False

c. Abscess formation has been associated in those with gonococcal infection. True/False

d. Abcesses and cysts can be treated conservatively. True/False

e. Surgical treatment involves abscess drainage and marsupialisation. True/False

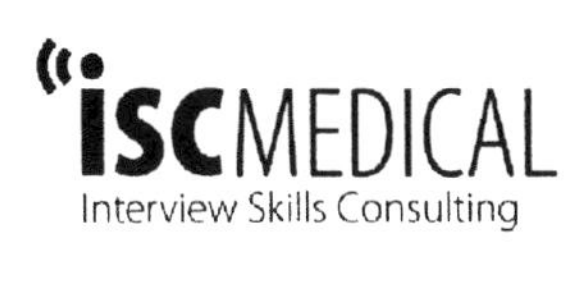

62 Vulval conditions. GYNAE

a. Vulval carcinoma is a squamous cell carcinoma. True/False

b. Vulval intraepithelial neoplasia (VIN) is associated with human papilloma virus. True/False

c. Lichen sclerosus can lead to carcinoma. True/False

d. VIN is a recurrent condition. True/False

e. Patients with recurrent vulval pain and itch can benefit from contact with the UK Vulval Pain Society. True/False

63 Pruritus vulvae can be caused by: GYNAE

a. Topical oestrogens. True/False

b. Leukoplakia. True/False

c. Threadworms. True/False

d. Lichen sclerosus. True/False

e. Renal failure. True/False

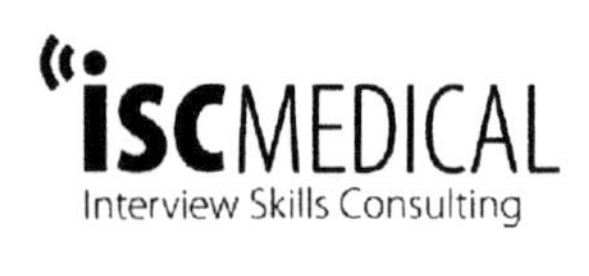

64 Hydatiform mole. **GYNAE**

a. Can mimic features of hyperthyroidism. True/False

b. Rarely leads to choriocarcinoma. True/False

c. Pregnancy should be avoided for 12 months after b-HCG levels are returned to normal following a complete mole. True/False

d. Oral contraceptive pill is contraindicated during active disease. True/False

e. Is associated with a risk of further ectopic pregnancy. True/False

65 Management of ectopic pregnancy. **GYNAE**

a. In acute decompensation, the patient should be taken straight to theatre. True/False

b. Laparotomy is superior to laparoscopy, since it allows a better approach to trophoblasts that are difficult to access. True/False

c. Inadequate surgery can lead to a persisting trophoblast which leads to further ectopic pregnancies. True/False

d. Salpingectomy is preferred to salpingotomy in a patient with no previous gynaecological anomalies. True/False

e. Salpingectomy leads to fewer intrauterine pregnancies than those having salpingotomy. True/False

66	The following are associated with ectopic pregnancy.	GYNAE

a. Bacterial Vaginosis. True/False

b. Previous ectopic pregnancy. True/False

c. Emergency contraception. True/False

d. Inflammatory bowel disease. True/False

e. Endometriosis. True/False

67	Ectopic pregnancy.	GYNAE

a. This accounts for almost 10% of all pregnancies. True/False

b. Can be excluded by a negative urine pregnancy test. True/False

c. Peritoneal pregnancies can progress into the third trimester. True/False

d. Should be suspected in any sexually active woman who has vaginal bleeding or pelvic pains, whether or not they have missed a period. True/False

e. The vast majority (>95%) occur in the fallopian tubes. True/False

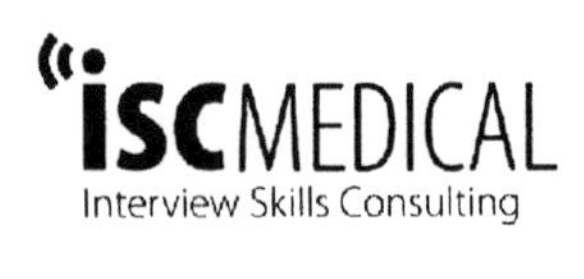

68	Recognised causes of recurrent spontaneous miscarriage are:	GYNAE

a. Migraine. True/False

b. Emergency contraception more than twice in the preceding year. True/False

c. Bacterial vaginosis. True/False

d. Vulvovaginal candidiasis. True/False

e. Cone biopsy for advanced cervical intraepithelial neoplasia. True/False

69	The following terms are correctly matched with their definitions.	GYNAE

a. Bleeding in early pregnancy which has resolved and the pregnancy continues : Missed abortion. True/False

b. Bleeding in early pregnancy where most of products of conception have been passed, but not all : Incomplete abortion. True/False

c. Bleeding in early pregnancy which later becomes a complete abortion : Threatened abortion. True/False

d. Early pregnancy vaginal bleeding where the foetus has died but not yet delivered : Inevitable abortion. True/False

e. Loss of 3 or more pregnancies : Recurrent spontaneous miscarriage. True/False

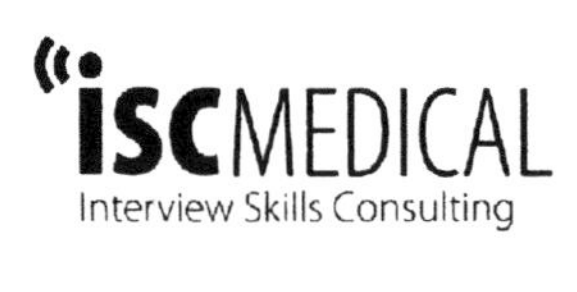

70 Pelvic inflammatory disease (PID). **GYNAE**

a. Most PID is caused by Chlamydia trachomatis. True/False

b. Should be treated as an inpatient with intravenous and oral antibiotics. True/False

c. Prompt treatment reduces the risk of subsequent tubal factor infertility. True/False

d. Increases the risk of ectopic pregnancy. True/False

e. Infertility risk increases with every episode of infection. True/False

71 The following may increase the risk of endometriosis. **GYNAE**

a. Oral contraceptive pill. True/False

b. Pregnancy. True/False

c. Intrauterine contraceptive device. True/False

d. Cervical cap. True/False

e. Family history. True/False

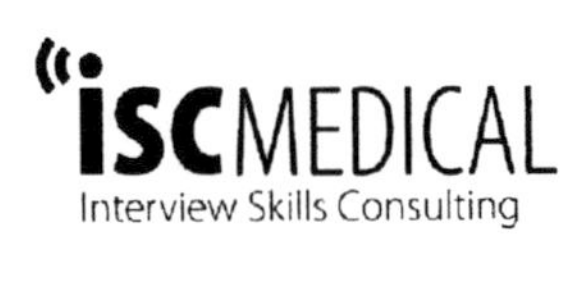

72 Regarding endometriosis. GYNAE

a. Most patients are treated with surgery. True/False

b. Medical treatments are hormonal and suppress ovulation, but lead to androgenic side effects. True/False

c. Deposits can be found beyond the peritoneal cavity. True/False

d. It is recognised to lead to preterm delivery. True/False

e. Affects up to 5% of women. True/False

73 The cervix. GYNAE

a. The transition zone is the point at which the inferior margin merges with the vaginal vault. True/False

b. Cervical polyps are benign and are treated conservatively. True/False

c. Nabothian cysts should be reviewed on a yearly basis. True/False

d. Cervical ectropion is a cause of post coital bleeding. True/False

e. Cervical ectropion can enlarge under hormonal influence. True/False

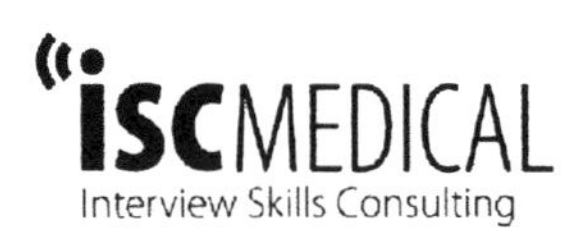

74	Subfertility.	GYNAE

a. Male factors account for about a quarter of cases. True/False

b. Serum progesterone around 21 days in cycle helps to confirm ovulation. True/False

c. A man should abstain from ejaculation for at least 3 days before semen analysis. True/False

d. Samples for semen analysis should be stored in a fridge if transport delay is anticipated. True/False

e. Hysterosalpingiogram is an essential first line investigation of the woman. True/False

75	Choriocarcinoma.	GYNAE

a. Is unlikely once a year has passed after a pregnancy. True/False

b. Can present with haemoptysis. True/False

c. Responds poorly to chemotherapy. True/False

d. Metastases are treated with excision or radiotherapy. True/False

e. Fertility can be maintained after successful treatment. True/False

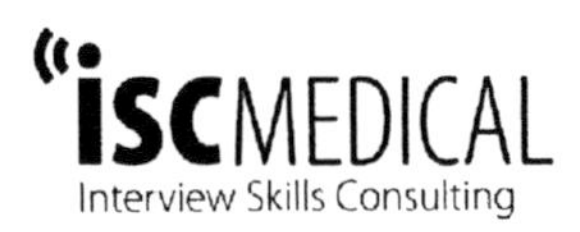

76 Treatment of subfertility. GYNAE

a. Artificial insemination by partner is useful when sperm count is low. True/False

b. Anovulation can be circumvented by high dose oestrogens. True/False

c. Hyperstimulation of the ovary by medication risks multiple pregnancies. True/False

d. Artificial insemination is contraindicated in HIV patients, whether they are donors or recipients. True/False

e. Each cycle of IVF has a success rate of around 10%. True/False

77 Non-hormonal contraception. GYNAE

a. Spermicides, if applied properly, can be used alone with reliable results. True/False

b. If well practiced, restricting coitus to certain days in the cycle can significantly reduce risk of pregnancy. True/False

c. Cervical caps can reduce the risk of gonococcal infection in the female. True/False

d. Pregnancy rate is practically zero if the male manages to ejaculate outside the vagina. True/False

e. The 'teat' on the end of the condom must be left open and not squeezed so that it can receive the semen otherwise the condom will burst. True/False

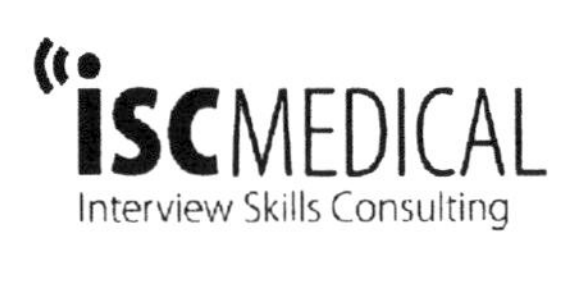

78 Intrauterine contraceptive device (IUD). GYNAE

a. Must be changed every 2 years. True/False

b. Works mainly by the direct toxic effect of copper on the spermatozoa, ova and blastocyst. True/False

c. Increases the long term risk of pelvic infection. True/False

d. The progesterone-carrying intrauterine system (IUS) can reduce problems of heavy periods. True/False

e. Pregnancy with an IUD in situ is likely to be ectopic. True/False

79 Emergency contraception. GYNAE

a. The progesterone-only emergency contraceptive (EC) is only useful until 24 hours after coitus. True/False

b. EC is contraindicated in those post sexual assault. True/False

c. An intrauterine contraceptive device can be used up until day 19 of a 28 day cycle. True/False

d. EC affects tubal motility and risks ectopic implantation and hence ectopic pregnancy. True/False

e. EC may be purchased over the counter (without prescription). True/False

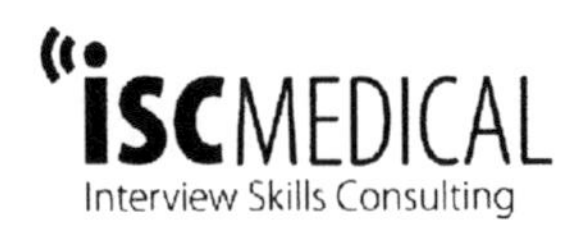

80	The following are absolute contraindications to the combined oral contraceptive pill.	GYNAE

a. As yet undiagnosed genital tract bleeding. True/False

b. Body Mass Index > 39kg/m2. True/False

c. Any single cardiac risk factor. True/False

d. Previous Hepatitis A. True/False

e. Porphyria. True/False

81	The combined oral contraceptive pill (COCP).	GYNAE

a. Those taking amoxycillin should be warned of reduced effectiveness of COCP and the need to use barrier contraception. True/False

b. When an enzyme inducing drug is taken at the same time, barrier methods should be advised for just the time at which the inducing drug is taken. True/False

c. COCP has a similar stroke risk to Progesterone only Pill (PoP). True/False

d. COCP is absolutely contraindicated in those with Migraine. True/False

e. Any increase risk of breast cancer is mainly in young women taking the COCP. True/False

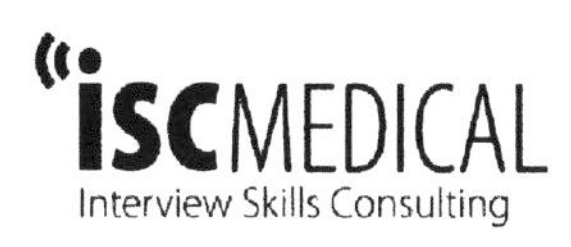

82	The progesterone-only pill (PoP).	GYNAE

a. Leads to erratic bleeding in many women. True/False

b. Most act by suppressing ovulation. True/False

c. Can be used in those with a chaotic lifestyle. True/False

d. Is not affected by diarrhoeal illnesses. True/False

e. Can be taken by those who are breastfeeding. True/False

83	Depot and implant hormonal contraception.	GYNAE

a. Depot injection is given 6 monthly. True/False

b. Depot injection is useful in a women on TB therapy. True/False

c. Depot often leads to temporary amenorrhoea. True/False

d. The implant will continue to provide a woman with contraception for up to 3 months after removal. True/False

e. Implants are changed yearly. True/False

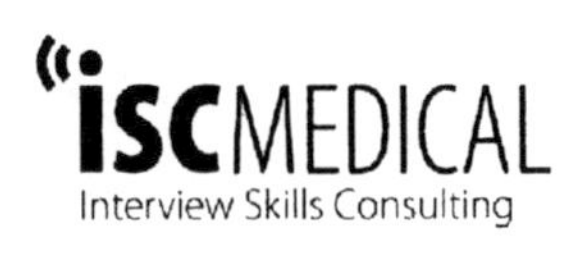

84	Contraceptive methods.	GYNAE

a. The combined oral contraceptive pill can be prescribed as a treatment for acne. True/False

b. Diaphragms come in just one size but can be stretched to fit the anatomical dimensions of any patient (posterior fornix to pubic bone). True/False

c. A young woman having regular sex without contraception has an 80% to 90% risk of pregnancy per year. True/False

d. Depot (injectable) progestogens are better than progestogens implants for those who may wish to conceive in a year's time because of the short half-life of the injected medication and rapid return to fertility. True/False

e. Progestogen-only pills are used in those who have a high risk of venous thromboembolism. True/False

85	Cervical screening.	GYNAE

a. Should routinely start at the age of 25. True/False

b. Moderate to severe dyskaryosis should be referred to colposcopy. True/False

c. The smear will tell what (if any) level of cervical intraepithelial neoplasia (CIN) is present. True/False

d. Screening can stop once a woman reaches 50. True/False

e. Given time, CIN 1, 2 and 3 after dormancy will progress to a higher stage and ultimately cancer. True/False

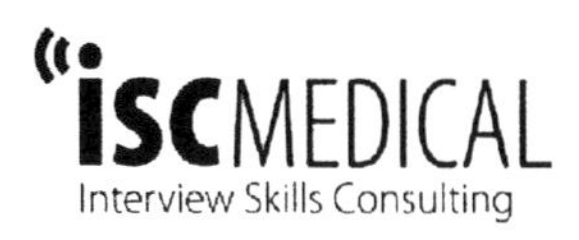

86	Abortion.	GYNAE

a. About 1 in 5 pregnancies miscarry. True/False

b. 10% of early miscarriages are due to intercurrent maternal illness. True/False

c. Bacterial vaginosis leads to first trimester abortions. True/False

d. Miscarriage due to cervical incompetence tends to present in the first trimester. True/False

e. Chronic medical diseases (e.g. diabetes) during pregnancy tend to lead to mid trimester abortions. True/False

87	Prolapse.	GYNAE

a. A urethrocele often leads to urge incontinence. True/False

b. Pelvic floor exercises help to prevent prolapse. True/False

c. Ring pessaries are sufficient in many to manage uterine prolapse. True/False

d. Weight loss is a strategy to resolve problems. True/False

e. Severe uterine prolapse can lead to cervical ulceration. True/False

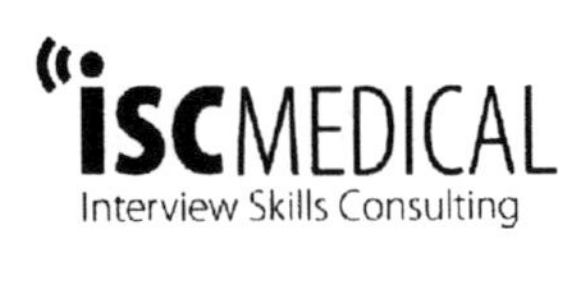

88	Polycystic ovarian syndrome.	GYNAE

a. Dianette® has a cosmetic use. True/False

b. Metformin is of value. True/False

c. It increases TIA & CVA rates by threefold. True/False

d. Hypertension is a recognised feature. True/False

e. Ultrasound is important in the diagnosis. True/False

89	The following are recognised risk factors for developing cervical carcinoma.	GYNAE

a. HIV. True/False

b. High number of sexual partners. True/False

c. High number of pregnancies. True/False

d. Late onset of sexual activity. True/False

e. Tobacco smoking. True/False

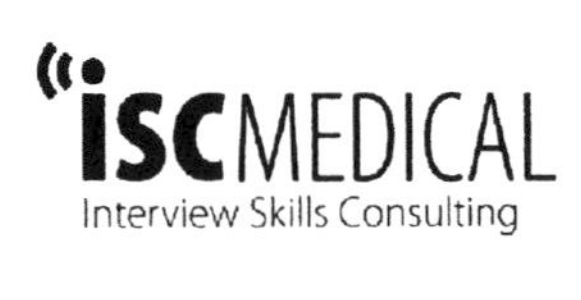

90 Termination of pregnancy (TOP). GYNAE

a. Medical abortion can be used up to 26 weeks of pregnancy. True/False

b. Up to 20% will require a surgical procedure following medical management. True/False

c. Patients under 18 years will require Gemeprost or misoprostil prior to surgical procedure. True/False

d. Mifepristone and Gemeprost for medical TOP can sometimes cause dysmenorrhoea and prolonged uterine contractions in the following days after TOP. True/False

e. Pre TOP ultrasound is always performed in order to exclude ectopic implantation or molar pregnancies. True/False

91 Termination of pregnancy (TOP). GYNAE

a. Must never be performed after 24 weeks. True/False

b. Must always have at least two doctors signing for it. True/False

c. Should involve an STI screen. True/False

d. Concurrent Chlamydia, if untreated, will cause a case of salpingitis for every 4 patients with it having a TOP. True/False

e. A doctor can refuse to sign for it and refer the patient to someone else. True/False

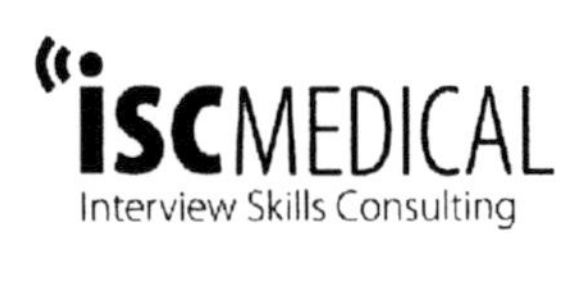

92 Hormone replacement therapy (HRT). **GYNAE**

a. Is acceptable to many as a patch containing both oestrogen and progesterone. True/False

b. The increased risk of breast cancer rises after the first year of use. True/False

c. Should be withheld in everyone with a family history of breast cancer. True/False

d. Therapy may need to be withheld if there is a past history of varicose veins. True/False

e. If using just topical vaginal gels of oestrogen, oral progestagens are not required. True/False

93 Ovarian carcinoma. **GYNAE**

a. May present with obstructive uropathy. True/False

b. Chemotherapy is curative in many cases. True/False

c. Has the greatest mortality out of all the gynaecological tumours. True/False

d. Is associated with breast carcinoma. True/False

e. Risks are reduced in those on the combined oral contraceptive. True/False

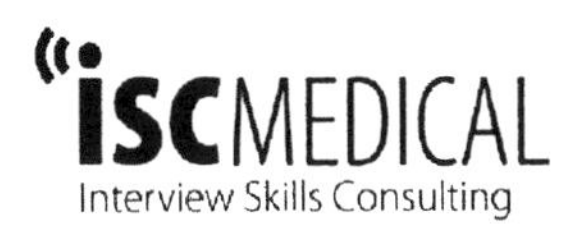

94	Hormone replacement therapy (HRT).	GYNAE

a. Can increase ovarian cancer risk. True/False

b. Should be given as oestrogen and progesterone if the woman has had a vaginal hysterectomy. True/False

c. Can reduce the risk of cardiovascular disease. True/False

d. May protect against dementia. True/False

e. Protects against osteomalacia. True/False

95	The following features are commonly associated with a hydatidiform mole.	GYNAE

a. A very high betaHCG. True/False

b. Abdominal pain. True/False

c. Excessive nausea and vomiting. True/False

d. Pelvic bleeding. True/False

e. 'Snowstorm' appearance on abdominal ultrasound. True/False

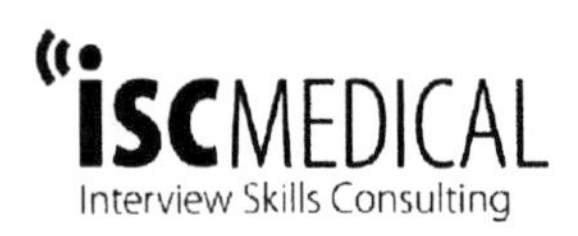

96 Cervical carcinoma. GYNAE

a. Carcinoma is most often detected from abnormal smears. True/False

b. Wertheim's hysterectomy is reserved for stage I tumours (confined to cervix). True/False

c. Sexual intercourse should be avoided for up to 3 months post radiotherapy. True/False

d. Repeat smears should be taken on a regular basis following chemo-radiotherapy. True/False

e. Glandular tissue on a smear result suggests adenocarcinoma of the cervix. True/False

97 Menorrhagia. GYNAE

a. Endometriosis and fibroids are most commonly the cause in young women. True/False

b. Mefanamic acid can help with the excessive blood loss. True/False

c. The combined oral contraceptive pill (COCP) is the treatment of choice for dysfunctional uterine bleeding (DUB) in women up to the age of 50. True/False

d. Hypothyroidism is a recognised cause. True/False

e. The Mirena ® intrauterine system is a first line treatment which can also reduce fibroid size. True/False

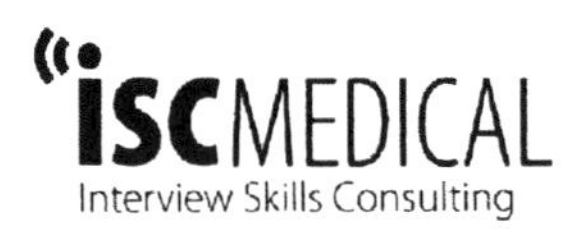

98 Contraindications to hormone replacement therapy include: **GYNAE**

a. Previous pulmonary embolus. True/False

b. Lupus nephritis. True/False

c. Hypertension. True/False

d. Being a smoker. True/False

e. Dubin-Johnson syndrome. True/False

99 Amenorrhoea. **GYNAE**

a. May be solved by karyotyping. True/False

b. Can be associated with galactorrhoea. True/False

c. Investigations should involve LH, Testosterone and TFTs. True/False

d. Psychotherapeutic treatment may be useful in some cases. True/False

e. Commonly leads to permanent infertility. True/False

100 Postmenopausal bleeding. **GYNAE**

a. Must be referred if it occurs after 6 months of last period. True/False

b. Must be considered due to endometrial carcinoma until proven otherwise. True/False

c. Can be related to HRT withdrawal. True/False

d. Is more common if the patient had an IUD. True/False

e. Can be caused by atrophic vaginitis. True/False

101 Postcoital bleeding. **GYNAE**

a. Cannot be due to cervical cancer if the patient is HPV negative. True/False

b. Is due to cervical neoplasia until proven otherwise. True/False

c. Is uncommon on the minipill. True/False

d. Is often seen in bacterial vaginosis. True/False

e. Is noted with trichomonas vaginalis. True/False

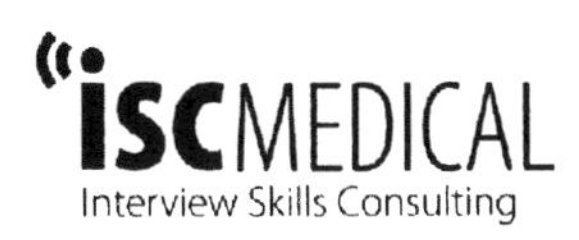

102 Secondary dysmenorrhoea. **GYNAE**

a. Means painful periods with heavy flow. True/False

b. Occurs straight from menarche without ever experiencing normal periods. True/False

c. Can be caused by chlamydial infection. True/False

d. Can be caused by TB. True/False

e. Is unlikely to be due to fibroids if patient is over 40 years of age. True/False

103 Primary dysmenorrhoea. **GYNAE**

a. Is due to overactive hormonal interaction with the corpus luteum. True/False

b. Is linked to polycystic ovarian syndrome. True/False

c. Responds well to paracetamol. True/False

d. Involves heavy bleeding. True/False

e. Prostaglandin inhibitors can be of benefit. True/False

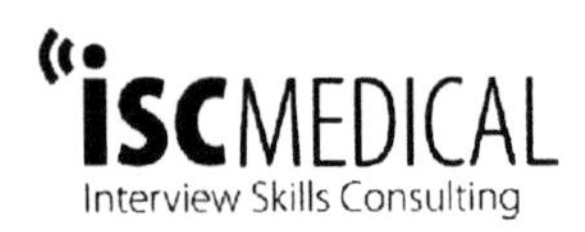

104 The menstrual cycle. **GYNAE**

a. Is 28 days in only 12% of women. True/False

b. FSH predominates in the first half. True/False

c. Cervical mucus is at its most receptive to sperm in the follicular stage. True/False

d. Oestrogen exerts a positive and negative feedback on the pituitary. True/False

e. The corpus luteum becomes the source of progesterone. True/False

105 A retroverted uterus. **GYNAE**

a. Occurs in 5% of all women. True/False

b. It leads to an increase in bowel disturbance especially in diverticular disease. True/False

c. Is commonly associated with dyspareunia. True/False

d. May lead to urinary retention in pregnancy. True/False

e. Associated with breech births. True/False

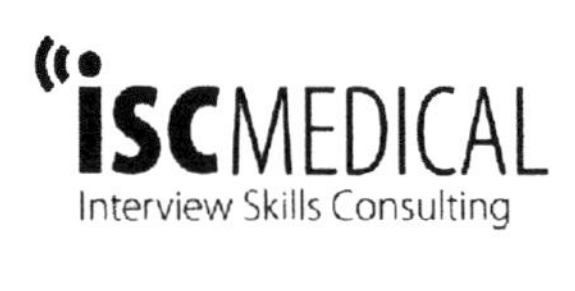

106 Treatments for premenstrual syndrome include the following: **GYNAE**

a. Mefanamic acid for energy and mood. True/False

b. Low fat diet for mastalgia. True/False

c. High protein diet for mood. True/False

d. Ginkgo Biloba for irritability. True/False

e. Bromocriptine for mastalgia. True/False

107 Ovarian tumours. **GYNAE**

a. Mucinous cystadenomas tend to lead to Meig's syndrome. True/False

b. Meigs' syndrome is when an ovarian tumour causes ascites. True/False

c. Pseudomyxoma peritonei can be caused by ovarian tumours which rupture and seed the peritoneum. True/False

d. Functional cysts are very common and in fact very small ones are regarded as normal. True/False

e. Out of all cysts, serous cysts are most likely to be malignant. True/False

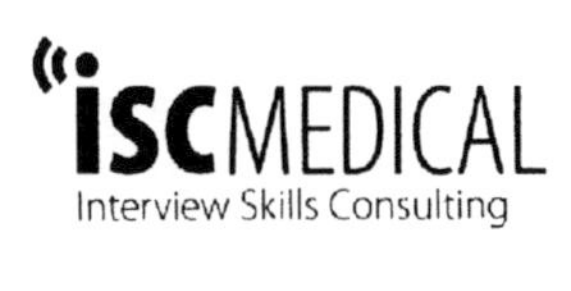

108 Menopause. **GYNAE**

a. Can be confused with thyroid dysfunction. True/False

b. Most symptoms result from lack of oestrogen action on the body. True/False

c. Vaginal dryness can lead to urinary tract infection. True/False

d. Raloxifene a selective oestrogen receptor modulator protects bones whilst reducing breast cancer risk and hot flushes. True/False

e. Hormone replacement is contraindicated in women who have had a hysterectomy. True/False

109 The following are recognised consequences of bacterial vaginosis. **GYNAE**

a. Reduced fertility. True/False

b. Preterm labour. True/False

c. Sepsis post termination of pregnancy. True/False

d. Increased chance of HIV acquisition. True/False

e. Ectopic pregnancy. True/False

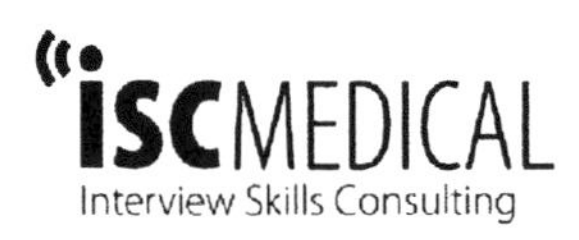

110 The following is true of bacterial vaginosis. **GYNAE**

a. Is less likely in a pH below 4.5. True/False

b. 'Clue cells' on microscopy are pathognomic. True/False

c. Partner treatment is also indicated. True/False

d. Is present in around 10% of women. True/False

e. Can be precipitated by unprotected sexual intercourse. True/False

111 The following are recognised causes of odorous vaginal discharge. **GYNAE**

a. Trichomonas vaginalis. True/False

b. Candida albicans. True/False

c. Bacterial vaginosis. True/False

d. Chlamydia trachomatis (serovars D to K). True/False

e. Neisseria gonococcus. True/False

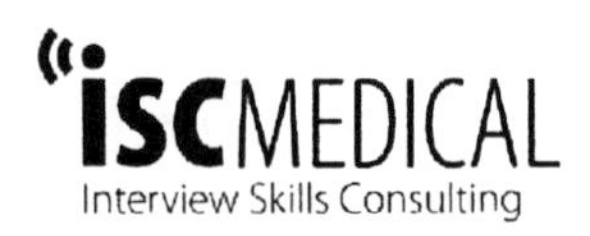

112 The following is true of ovarian tumours. **GYNAE**

a. Over 90% are benign (cysts). True/False

b. Combined oral contraceptive is protective against carcinomas. True/False

c. Ovulatory induction agents in infertility treatments are a risk for malignancy. True/False

d. Malignant tumours are associated with the BRCA (breast carcinoma) gene types. True/False

e. High fat intake increases risk of malignancy. True/False

113 The following are associated with an increased risk of endometrial carcinoma. **GYNAE**

a. Obesity. True/False

b. Multiparity. True/False

c. Tamoxifen. True/False

d. Diabetes. True/False

e. Polycystic ovaries. True/False

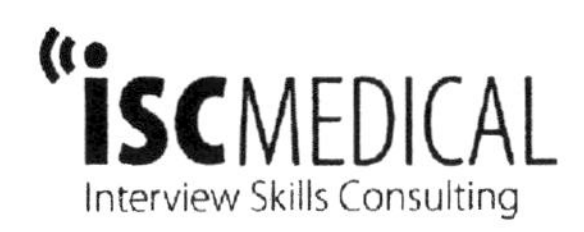

114 Treatment of fibroids. **GYNAE**

a. Irregularities of bleeding respond best to oral hormonal contraceptives. True/False

b. Most women eventually require medical or surgical therapies. True/False

c. Red degeneration can lead to rapid decompensation hence necessitating urgent surgical intervention. True/False

d. Most fibroids affect the body of the uterus and so expansion in pregnancy does not always lead to a caesarean section. True/False

e. Fibroids can be treated by radiologically guided injection of an embolising agent. True/False

115 Complications of fibroids include: **GYNAE**

a. Deep vein thrombosis. True/False

b. Pelvic inflammatory disease. True/False

c. Choriocarcinoma. True/False

d. Urinary frequency. True/False

e. Obstruction to labour. True/False

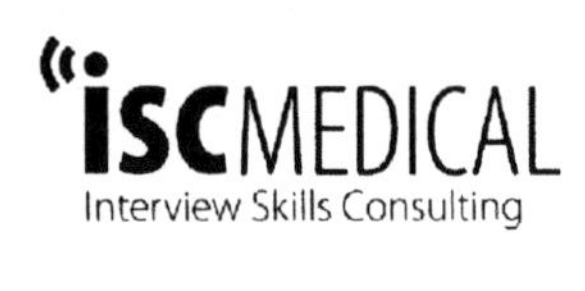

116 Fibroids. **GYNAE**

a. Tend to atrophy in the menopause. True/False

b. Are more common in smokers. True/False

c. Occur in at least 20% of women. True/False

d. Commonly shrink during pregnancy. True/False

e. Increasing size of a fibroid in a postmenopausal woman should suggest a malignant change. True/False

117 The following are recognised precipitants to endometritis. **GYNAE**

a. Childbirth. True/False

b. IUCD insertion. True/False

c. Allergy to latex condoms. True/False

d. Ulcerative colitis. True/False

e. Nabothian cysts. True/False

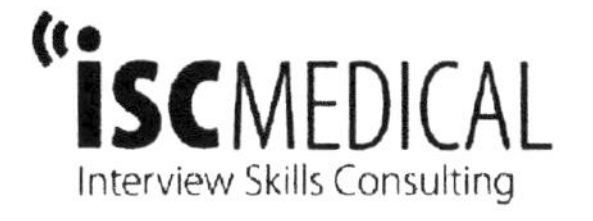

MCQs for GPVTS

OBSTETRICS

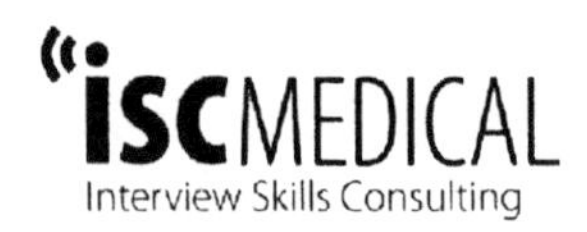

118 The following are recognised risk factors for the development of pre-eclampsia. **OBS**

a. Alcohol consumption during pregnancy. True/False

b. Anticonvulsant medications. True/False

c. Sexual relationship of partner less than 3 months. True/False

d. Past history of migraine. True/False

e. Iron deficiency anaemia. True/False

119 Induction of labour. **OBS**

a. Cervical ripeness is assessed by scoring several features including size and consistency. True/False

b. Induction is contraindicated in a breech presentation. True/False

c. A cervix can ripen under the influence of topical steroids. True/False

d. Prostaglandins are used in induction but can only work on a ripe cervix. True/False

e. Once the cervix begins to dilate, the membranes will soon rupture. Artificial rupture should be avoided if possible since this risks ascending infection. True/False

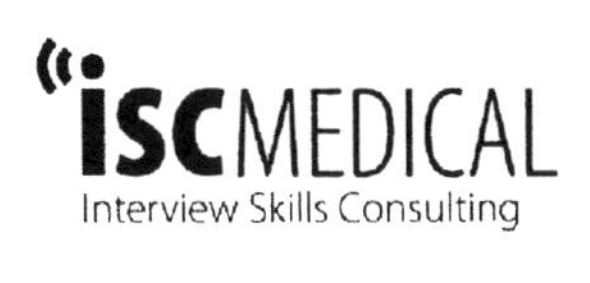

120 The following is true regarding toxoplasmosis. **OBS**

a. Typically causes meningitis in the neonate. True/False

b. If diagnosed in the pregnant woman, the risk to her baby has already peaked and no effective treatment can given. True/False

c. Foetal IgM diagnoses foetal acquisition. True/False

d. In pregnant women, presentation can resemble a glandular fever type syndrome. True/False

e. Risk is reduced by avoiding gardening. True/False

121 The following is true regarding polyhydramnios. **OBS**

a. Is suggested by increased abdominal girth in the pregnant mother. True/False

b. Predisposes towards premature delivery. True/False

c. Predisposes towards cord prolapse. True/False

d. Prostaglandins can reduce foetal urine production and temporarily relieve problems. True/False

e. It is defined as amniotic fluid greater than 1 litre in volume. True/False

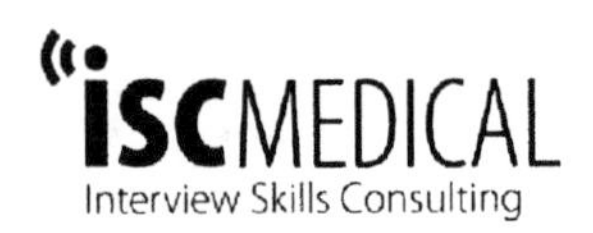

122 The following features in a pregnant woman with BP >140/90 mmHg and proteinuria necessitate urgent delivery. **OBS**

a. Pruritis. True/False

b. Visual disturbance. True/False

c. Headache. True/False

d. Urinary frequency. True/False

e. Platelets < 100x10^9/l. True/False

123 The following is true regarding pre-eclampsia. **OBS**

a. Risk is reduced by taking aspirin. True/False

b. Pre-eclampsia may develop from the 20th week onwards. True/False

c. Pre-eclampsia is asymptomatic. If symptoms present, this is termed eclampsia. True/False

d. Beta blockers have a role to play in prevention. True/False

e. Its pathogenesis involves maternal sensitisation to small amounts of foetal antigens which leak into the maternal circulation causing a non-specific cytokine response resulting in hypertension with liver and renal effects. True/False

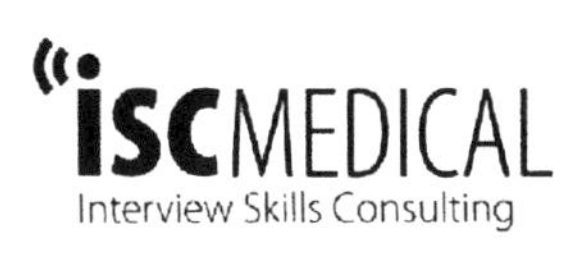

124 The following is true regarding the management of pre-eclampsia and eclampsia. **OBS**

a. Delivery removes risk from pre-eclampsia and sinister sequelae only occur up until about an hour postpartum. True/False

b. H2 blockers should be given routinely. True/False

c. Magnesium sulphate levels must be monitored since high levels are toxic. True/False

d. Fluid restriction is often necessary. True/False

e. Steroids play a role in delaying complications while theatre is being prepared for caesarean section. True/False

125 Foetal monitoring. **OBS**

a. Kick charts suggest foetal distress when more than 12 kicks are registered per day. True/False

b. Cardiotocography (CTG) measures uterine contractions along with foetal heart rate. True/False

c. Foetal bradycardia is often associated with hypoxia in the foetus. True/False

d. Beat to beat variability is a normal sign that is expected on a CTG in labour. True/False

e. Late decelerations reflect impairment of foetal vagal responses and suggest hypoxia. True/False

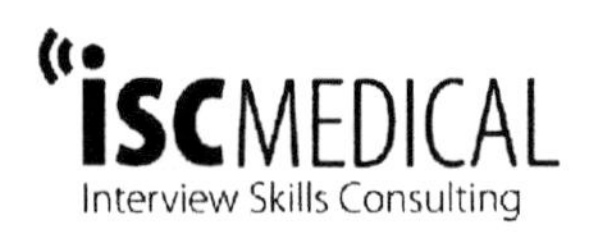

126 The following is true regarding rubella and pregnancy. **OBS**

a. Antenatal rubella screening identifies those who require vaccination before delivery. True/False

b. Infection in most pregnant women is asymptomatic. True/False

c. Is associated with cataracts in the newborn. True/False

d. Is associated with ophthalmia neonatorum. True/False

e. The risk of problems to the foetus is the greatest in the first trimester. True/False

127 The following is true regarding pre-eclampsia and eclampsia. **OBS**

a. Maternal death is often due to accelerated phase hypertension and heart failure. True/False

b. Patients with a rise in blood pressure > 30/20 mmHg should be admitted. True/False

c. Magnesium sulphate has a role in terminating seizures. True/False

d. Beta blockers are contraindicated in managing hypertension. True/False

e. Ergometrine is contraindicated during labour. True/False

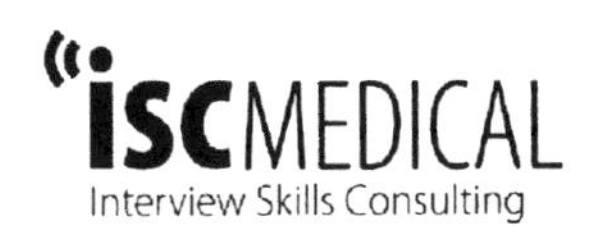

128 The following is true regarding sexually transmitted infections and pregnancy. **OBS**

a. Syphilis in a pregnant women with no drug allergies should be treated with a 10 day course of intramuscular penicillin. True/False

b. Maternal Chlamydia trachomatis can lead to a pneumonitis in the neonate. True/False

c. Herpes simplex virus acquired before conception poses a negligible risk to the neonate if lesions are not present at time of delivery. True/False

d. Genital warts tend to be resistant to treatment during pregnancy. True/False

e. Genital warts during pregnancy pose an extremely low risk of papilloma in the neonate. True/False

129 Premature rupture of membranes. **OBS**

a. A positive result on a nitrazine stick sampled from the high vagina gives definite confirmation of membrane rupture. True/False

b. The majority of cases will go on to labour. True/False

c. Delaying delivery is advantageous since it reduces the risk of ascending infection. True/False

d. Sepsis is a significant cause for premature rupture of membranes. True/False

e. Antibiotics given to the mother with premature rupture of membranes reduce the risk of intraventricular haemorrhage in the preterm neonate. True/False

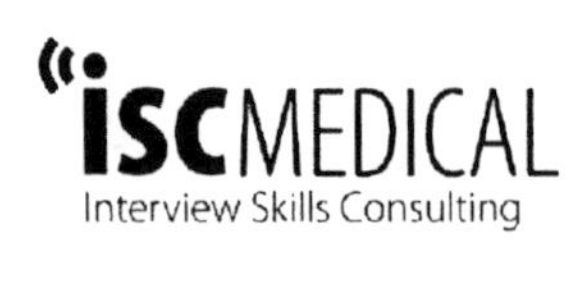

130 The following is true regarding analgesia during labour. **OBS**

a. Epidural anaesthesia is contraindicated in any woman receiving subcutaneous heparin therapy during labour. True/False

b. Pudendal nerve block is insufficient analgesia if rotational forceps are to be used. True/False

c. Epidurals lead to an increased risk of urinary incontinence during labour. True/False

d. Pethidine should not be given if delivery is expected with 2 hours. True/False

e. Intravenous fluid infusion is required during epidural anaesthesia. True/False

131 Management of preterm labour. **OBS**

a. Contractions may spontaneously stop in about half of cases. True/False

b. Steroids are of no significant value to the neonate if beyond 34 weeks gestation. True/False

c. Treating underlying cause e.g. sepsis will settle the majority of contractions and revert preterm labour. True/False

d. Once the cervix is > 4 cm dilated then labour is unlikely to be averted. True/False

e. Steroids are of best benefit to the neonate if given within 12 hours of delivery. True/False

132 Foetal distress. **OBS**

a. Is implicated if the foetal pH> 7.4. True/False

b. Is suggested by the early passage of meconium. True/False

c. Is confirmed by low oxygen saturation on the foetal scalp electrode. True/False

d. Is suggested by a variable baseline in the foetal heart tracing. True/False

e. Is suggested by rapid foetal limb movements. True/False

133 Postmaturity. **OBS**

a. Is associated with twin birth. True/False

b. Is defined as delivery beyond the 40th gestational week. True/False

c. Is associated with an increased risk of stillbirth. True/False

d. Is associated with an increased risk of meconium aspiration. True/False

e. Dry skin in the neonate is commonly observed. True/False

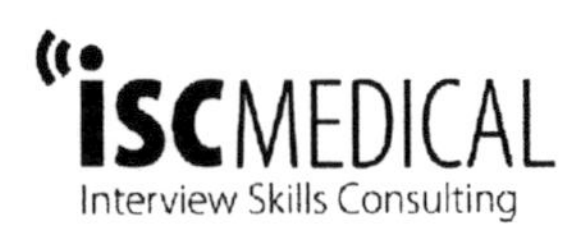

134	The following increase the risk of polyhydramnios.	OBS

a. Maternal hypothyroidism. True/False

b. Foetal duodenal atresia. True/False

c. Multiple pregnancy. True/False

d. Maternal hypertension. True/False

e. Maternal diabetes mellitus. True/False

135	The following tests form part of routine antenatal care in the UK.	OBS

a. Sickle cell tests if woman is black. True/False

b. Serum folate. True/False

c. HIV test. True/False

d. Syphilis test. True/False

e. Alphafetoprotein. True/False

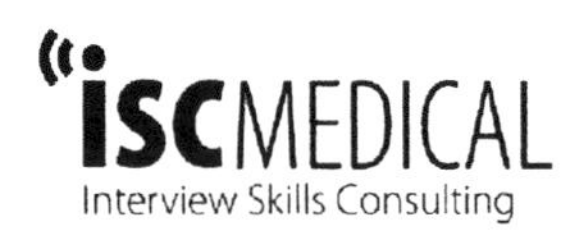

136 The following features of antepartum haemorrhage suggest placental abruption rather than placenta previa as the cause. **OBS**

a. No pain. True/False

b. Pre-eclampsia. True/False

c. Minimal visible blood loss. True/False

d. Small warning bleeds. True/False

e. Disseminated intravascular coagulation. True/False

137 The following are contraindications to tocolytic agents. **OBS**

a. Entonox True/False

b. Asthma. True/False

c. Premature rupture of membranes. True/False

d. Chorioamnionitis. True/False

e. Foetal death. True/False

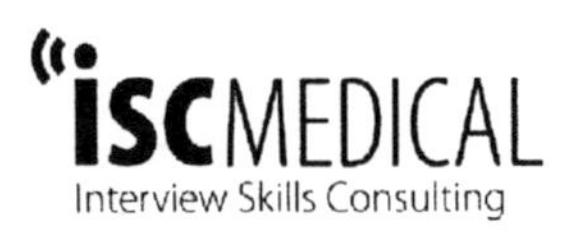

138	Coagulation disorders in pregnancy.	OBS

a. DIC is associated with trophoblastic disease. True/False

b. Acute fatty liver of pregnancy is associated with DIC. True/False

c. DIC is a complication of Rhesus disease during pregnancy. True/False

d. Maternal autoimmune thrombocytopenia purpura increases the risk of foetal intracranial haemorrhage around delivery. True/False

e. Maternal thrombocytopenia can be caused by folate deficiency. True/False

139	The following factors are recognised as increasing the chance of twin pregnancy.	OBS

a. Smoking. True/False

b. Uterine fibroids. True/False

c. Teenage pregnancy. True/False

d. Polycystic ovarian syndrome. True/False

e. Previous pelvic inflammatory disease. True/False

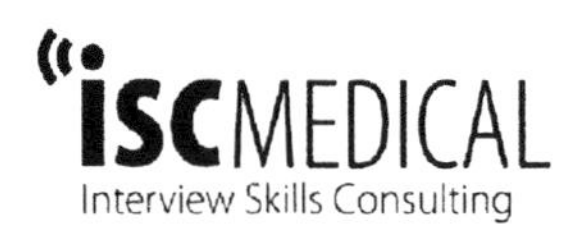

140 Hyperemesis gravidarum. **OBS**

a. Occurs in about 1% of pregnancies. True/False

b. May respond to an exclusion diet. True/False

c. Wernicke's encephalopathy is a recognised complication. True/False

d. Is associated with thyroid dysfunction. True/False

e. Is more common with a female foetus. True/False

141 Breech presentations. **OBS**

a. Most breech births present with the feet first (footling breech). True/False

b. Elective caesarean sections result in better outcomes than vaginal deliveries. True/False

c. External cephalic version (ECV) at 28 to 32 weeks has a roughly 50% success rate in turning the foetus. True/False

d. Anti D must be given to Rh D -ve women after ECV attempted. True/False

e. Forceps are invariably required for vaginal delivery. True/False

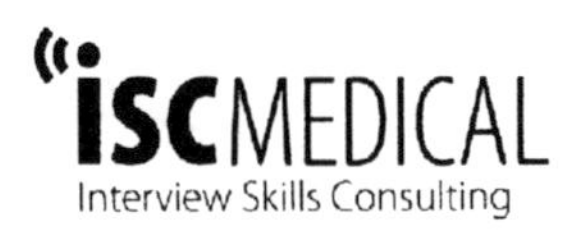

142 The following are indications for vertical incision approach to caesarean section. **OBS**

a. Maternal HIV seropositivity. True/False

b. BMI > 30 kg/m2. True/False

c. Placental abruption. True/False

d. Uterine fibroids. True/False

e. Recurrence of genital herpes at labour. True/False

143 Mendelson's syndrome. **OBS**

a. Prophylactic medications to reduce bronchospasm have a role in management. True/False

b. Proton pump inhibitors prior to anaesthetic are used to reduce gastric acid secretion and the limit the caustic effects of aspiration. True/False

c. Risk is reduced by preoperative intravenous sodium citrate. True/False

d. Emptying of the stomach prior to endotracheal intubation helps to reduce the incidence of this syndrome. True/False

e. Prophylactic antibiotics are routinely given to the mother. True/False

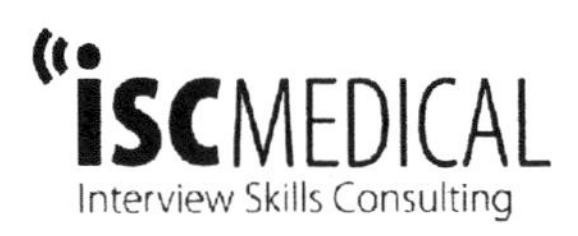

144 Uterine rupture. **OBS**

a. Minimal or absent per vaginal bleeding makes the diagnosis of a ruptured uterus unlikely. True/False

b. The majority of spontaneous ruptures will require hysterectomy. True/False

c. Forceps delivery increases the risk of uterine rupture. True/False

d. Previous cervical surgery increases the risk of uterine rupture. True/False

e. Use of steroids increases the risk of uterine rupture. True/False

145 The following are recognised causes of abdominal pain during pregnancy. **OBS**

a. Pre-eclampsia. True/False

b. Endometriosis. True/False

c. Uterine fibroids. True/False

d. Ovarian cysts. True/False

e. Uterine torsion. True/False

146 Stillbirth and death in utero. **OBS**

a. Stillbirth refers only to babies that die during labour and delivery. True/False

b. If labour doesn't ensue in utero death, it should be induced with amniotomy, prostaglandins and oxytocin. True/False

c. Induced labour following death in utero should be within 1 or 2 days to avoid significant risk of DIC after this point. True/False

d. Post mortem is a statutory obligation after still birth under UK law. True/False

e. No cause is found in up to a fifth of all cases of stillbirth. True/False

147 The following increase the risk of post partum haemorrhage. **OBS**

a. Young mother. True/False

b. Use of halothane anaesthesia. True/False

c. Twin birth. True/False

d. First pregnancy. True/False

e. Uterine fibroids. True/False

148 Retained placenta. **OBS**

a. May require hysterectomy if the placenta does not deliver with other extraction methods. True/False

b. Can be due to uterine atony. True/False

c. Is associated with the use of pethidine during labour. True/False

d. Is more common with twin births. True/False

e. Delivery of the placenta can be aided by the mother beginning to breast feed. True/False

149 Amniocentesis. **OBS**

a. Anti-D should be given to Rh D-ve women after the procedure. True/False

b. Is useful to gain foetal material for karyotyping. True/False

c. Is contraindicated if there is placenta previa. True/False

d. Can lead to miscarriage in up to 1 in 20 cases. True/False

e. Can be performed at an earlier stage in pregnancy than chorionic villous sampling. True/False

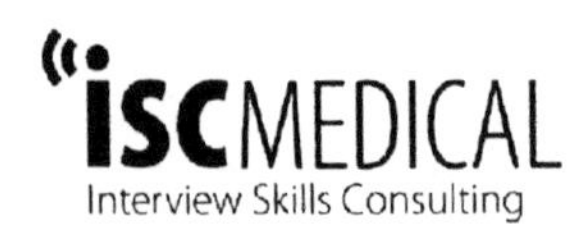

150	Amniotic fluid emboli.	OBS

a. They most often present during labour. True/False

b. Can occur as a complication to amniotic fluid sampling. True/False

c. Fluid resuscitation is contraindicated due to the high risk of pulmonary oedema in the mother. True/False

d. Diagnosis is confirmed by bronchoalveolar lavage of the mother revealing presence of foetal squamous cells. True/False

e. DIC is a recognised complication. True/False

151	The following are recognised complications of twin pregnancy.	OBS

a. Postmaturity. True/False

b. Polyhydramnios. True/False

c. Uterine rupture. True/False

d. Cord prolapse. True/False

e. Placenta previa. True/False

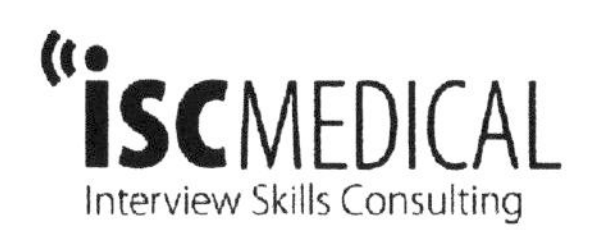

152 Rheumatological disease in pregnancy. **OBS**

a. SLE increases the risk of pre-eclampsia. True/False

b. Rheumatological conditions can lead to congenital heart block in the newborn. True/False

c. Antiphospholipid syndrome typically causes foetal loss in the third trimester. True/False

d. Antiphospholipid syndrome requires daily aspirin treatment to the mother. True/False

e. The risk of post partum DVT is increased in antiphospholipid syndrome. True/False

153 The following maternal conditions are modulated during pregnancy as stated below. **OBS**

a. Rheumatoid arthritis worsens during pregnancy. True/False

b. The majority of pregnant women with epilepsy have no increase or have a decrease in seizure frequency. True/False

c. Multiple sclerosis typically relapses during pregnancy. True/False

d. Hepatitis E carries an increased risk of mortality if the woman is pregnant rather than non-pregnant. True/False

e. Genital warts are recalcitrant to treatment during pregnancy. True/False

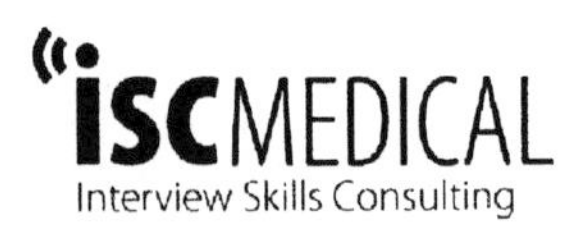

154 The following is true regarding jaundice during pregnancy. **OBS**

a. Vitamin K has to be given to the newborn. True/False

b. Ursodeoxycholic acid is contraindicated. True/False

c. Acute hepatosteatosis is an indication to expedite delivery. True/False

d. The incidence of gallstones is very low during pregnancy. True/False

e. Those with Gilbert's syndrome are at greater risk of dangerous jaundice and so bilirubin must be closely monitored. True/False

155 The following is true regarding birth injuries. **OBS**

a. Moulding is the term for compression or distortion of the foetal head during delivery and is associated with significant risk of intracranial haemorrhage. True/False

b. Cephalhaematoma is a subperiosteal swelling. True/False

c. Cephalhaematoma may take a few weeks to reabsorb. True/False

d. Caput succedaneum is a soft tissue swelling superior to the cranial bones and is more common with ventouse delivery. True/False

e. Subaponeurotic haematoma is often slow to reabsorb and since many are at risk of necrosis and infection, surgical drainage is often indicated. True/False

156 Perineal tears and episiotomy. **OBS**

a. Tears to the labia almost rarely require suturing. True/False

b. Tears are less common with forceps delivery. True/False

c. Second degree tears involve the rectal mucosa. True/False

d. Third degree tears are very likely to require epidural or general anaesthesia for repair. True/False

e. Rectal diclofenac is advisable postpartum following episiotomy. True/False

157 The puerperium. **OBS**

a. Expression of milk must continue in the event of mastitis or breast abscess. True/False

b. Lochia is expected to remain red for around 3 days post partum. True/False

c. Colostrum persists for a week post partum. True/False

d. The external cervical os typically remains open for about 3 weeks. True/False

e. The uterus takes on average 3 weeks to shrink back to remain a pelvic organ. True/False

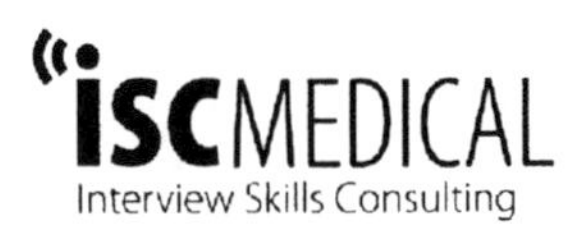

158 Heart disease and pregnancy. **OBS**

a. Cardioversion for tachyarrhythmias is contraindicated. True/False

b. Ampicillin and gentamicin is a recommended regimen during labour for women with heart valve disease. True/False

c. An ejection systolic murmur is normal in the vast majority of women. True/False

d. The lithotomy position is best avoided for delivery in pregnant patients with cardiac failure. True/False

e. A third heart sound is normal in the majority of women. True/False

159 The following is true regarding maternal diabetes mellitus. **OBS**

a. Along with ultrasound scanning, a foetal echocardiogram is commonly undertaken in pregnant women who have diabetes. True/False

b. Diabetic pregnant women are often admitted if glucose control at home is not optimal. True/False

c. Glycosuria during pregnancy is common and not often due to maternal diabetes mellitus. True/False

d. Oral hypoglycaemics are best avoided during pregnancy. True/False

e. Insulin needs in the mother often decline with the increased glucose consumption by the foetus. True/False

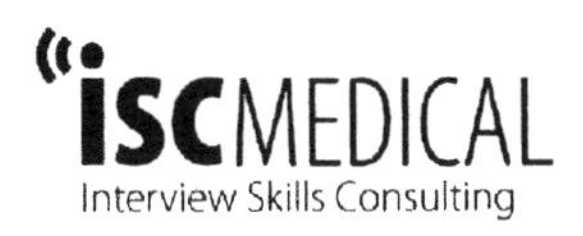

160 The following are recognised complications to the baby associated with diabetes mellitus in a pregnant woman. **OBS**

a. Intrauterine growth retardation. True/False

b. Neonatal biliary atresia. True/False

c. Polyhydramnios. True/False

d. Neonatal jaundice. True/False

e. Neonatal respiratory distress syndrome. True/False

161 Diabetes and pregnancy. **OBS**

a. Intravenous insulin by 'sliding scale' infusion is often used during labour. True/False

b. Insulin requirements fall during labour. True/False

c. Oral hypoglycaemics must not be reinstituted soon after birth. True/False

d. Gestational diabetes is associated with an increased risk of developing diabetes in later life. True/False

e. The majority of pregnant women found to have gestational diabetes will not develop diabetes in later life. True/False

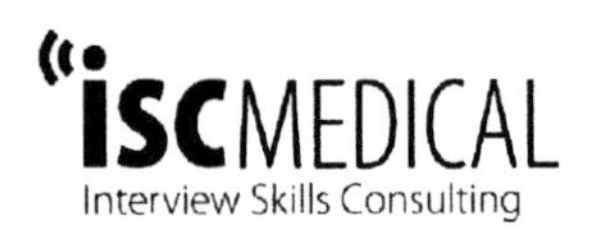

162 Thyroid disease and pregnancy. **OBS**

a. Hypothyroidism is more common than hyperthyroidism. True/False

b. Antithyroid drugs can be given during pregnancy and breast feeding. True/False

c. Radioactive iodine is contraindicated in pregnancy but safe in breast feeding. True/False

d. The severity of hyperthyroidism often falls during pregnancy. True/False

e. Postpartum thyroiditis is a relatively common condition. True/False

163 The following is true regarding uterine inversion. **OBS**

a. It occurs in about 5% of deliveries. True/False

b. Is associated with cord traction for a retained placenta. True/False

c. Halothane anaesthesia is useful during reversion. True/False

d. Is easily reverted with manual techniques by the delivery attendant. True/False

e. Prophylactic antibiotics are used after reversion. True/False

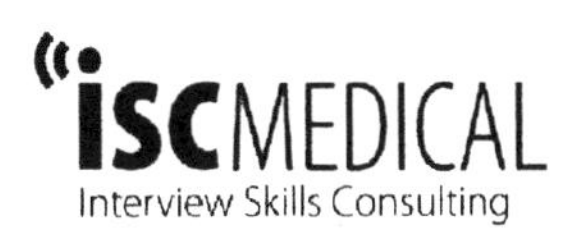

164 The following is true regarding problems during pregnancy. **OBS**

a. Reflux oesophagitis is often due to sphincter muscle relaxation. True/False

b. Around half of all women experience nausea and vomiting during pregnancy. True/False

c. Ankle oedema is rare in young women and often suggests proteinuria with pre-eclampsia. True/False

d. Pruritis in pregnancy may be the first sign of deranged liver functions and should be monitored carefully. True/False

e. Crampy leg or calf pain should not be dismissed, it is often a sign of deep vein thrombosis. True/False

165 The following is true regarding the use of forceps during labour. **OBS**

a. They can result in bruising and 'chignon' to the foetus. True/False

b. Their use is contraindicated with maternal pre-eclampsia. True/False

c. They aid delivery in cases when full cervical dilatation is not achieved. True/False

d. Their use is contraindicated in cases of cord prolapse. True/False

e. The bladder must be emptied prior to use. True/False

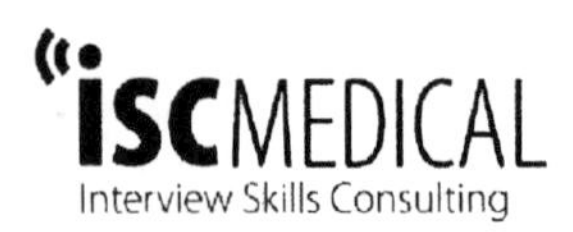

166	The following are indications for subcutaneous heparin administration following vaginal delivery.	OBS

a. Pre-eclampsia in a woman over 35 years of age. True/False

b. Labour lasting more than 12 hours in a woman weighing 90kg. True/False

c. Air travel during third trimester of pregnancy. True/False

d. Hypothyroidism. True/False

e. Antiphospholipid syndrome. True/False

167	The following shorthand is correctly matched with its definitions.	OBS

a. Para 2 + 0, gravida 3 : A woman who has been pregnant 3 times, with 2 deliveries and one terminated before 28 weeks. True/False

b. Gravida 3 : A woman who has been pregnant 3 times previously regardless of any current pregnancy. True/False

c. Para 2 + 1 : A woman has been pregnant 3 times. She had 2 full term deliveries and one which was delivered preterm but after 28 weeks. True/False

d. Para 2 gravida 2 : A woman who has had 2 pregnancies , no terminations and is currently not pregnant. True/False

e. Para 2 + 1 : A woman has been pregnant twice with one delivery beyond 28 weeks and one miscarriage before 28 weeks. True/False

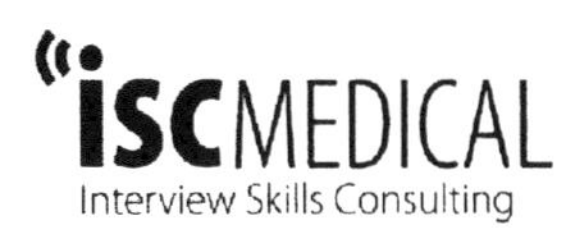

168	The following is true regarding 'normal' biochemistry reference ranges during pregnancy.	OBS

a. The upper limit of sodium range is reduced. True/False

b. The upper limit of calcium range is reduced. True/False

c. The alkaline phosphatase upper limit is increased. True/False

d. The urea upper limit rises. True/False

e. The creatinine upper limit rises. True/False

169	The following are recognised associations with placenta previa.	OBS

a. Assisted conception. True/False

b. Previous caesarian section. True/False

c. Uterine fibroids. True/False

d. Previous intrauterine contraceptive device. True/False

e. Multiple (e.g. twin) pregnancy. True/False

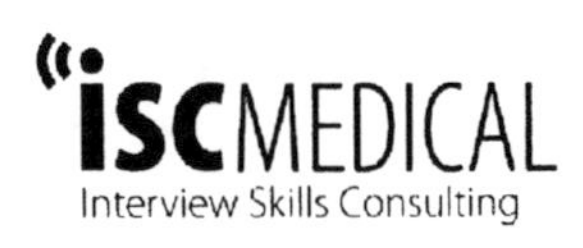

170 The following is true regarding uterine contractions. **OBS**

a. They commence at the fundus and spread out inferiorly. True/False

b. Dysfunctional contractions can be treated with oxytocin. True/False

c. Normally occur at a rate of 1 every two minutes. True/False

d. Can be enhanced by adrenaline. True/False

e. Are inhibited by analgesia. True/False

171 In an ideal pelvis, the following foetal presentations at birth are high risk for failure to progress during labour and often require caesarean section. **OBS**

a. Transverse lie. True/False

b. Flexed vertex. True/False

c. Occipitoposterior. True/False

d. Face. True/False

e. Occipitoanterior. True/False

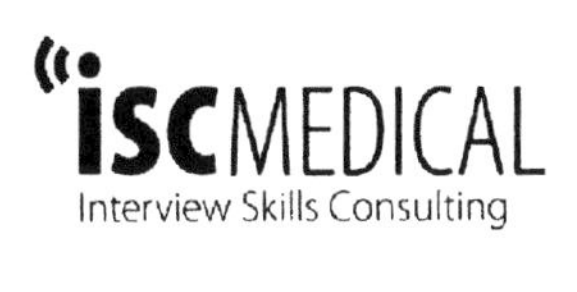

172 Gestational age and clinical assessment. **OBS**

a. The measurement from the symphisis pubis to the uterine fundus in inches (SFH) is used to estimate gestational age. True/False

b. An SFH of 38 at 32 weeks may be caused by maternal smoking. True/False

c. An SFH of 26 at 27 weeks is suggestive of poor intrauterine development. True/False

d. An SFH of 40 at 37 weeks is unremarkable. True/False

e. An SFH of 29 at 26 weeks is compatible with a twin pregnancy. True/False

173 Regarding the used of syntometrine in labour. **OBS**

a. This is used to induce labour when a pregnancy is overdue. True/False

b. This contains oxytocin. True/False

c. It is contraindicated in those with ischaemic heart disease. True/False

d. It has decreased the incidence of post partum haemorrhage. True/False

e. Can be used to hasten the third stage of labour as the shoulder of the neonate is presented at the introitus. True/False

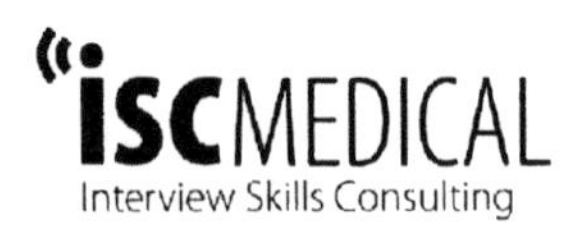

174 The following are associated with increased risk of hyperemesis gravidarum. **OBS**

a. Smoking. True/False

b. Multiple pregnancy. True/False

c. Pre-eclampsia. True/False

d. Age over 30. True/False

e. Hiatus hernia. True/False

175 The following is true regarding a normal labour. **OBS**

a. 'Cord lengthening' in the third stage implies detachment of the cord from the placenta and risk of retained products. True/False

b. Delivery of the anterior shoulder is aided by upward movement and rotation of the baby's head by the birth attendant. True/False

c. Second stage can vary in time between 15 minutes to 2 hours. True/False

d. The first stage of labour in a primip is expected to take around 12 hours. True/False

e. Crowning refers to the situation when the baby's head reaches the vulval aperture and the perineum stretches at this point. True/False

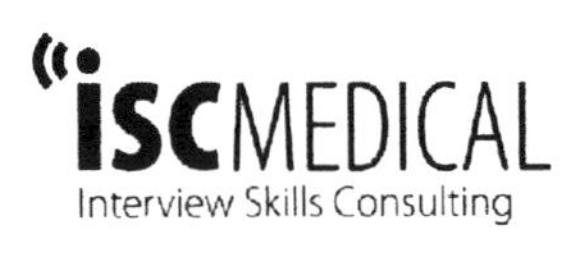

176 The following measurements are required during normal labour. **OBS**

a. Assess the rate and strength of contractions every 15 minutes. True/False

b. Vaginal examination to assess cervical dilatation every hour during the first stage. True/False

c. Test the mother's urine every 4 hours for the presence of ketones and protein. True/False

d. Measure the foetal heart rate every 30 minutes. True/False

e. Measure maternal vital signs every hour. True/False

177 Pregnancy tests. **OBS**

a. A urinary pregnancy test turns positive beyond 14 days from fertilisation. True/False

b. A negative pregnancy test 6 days after expected ovulation can rule out pregnancy. True/False

c. A pregnancy test will remain positive until the third trimester of most pregnancies. True/False

d. Urinary Beta HCG in contrast to serum HCG is specific for pregnancy and is negative in trophoblastic disease. True/False

e. Remains positive for up to 5 days after an abortion. True/False

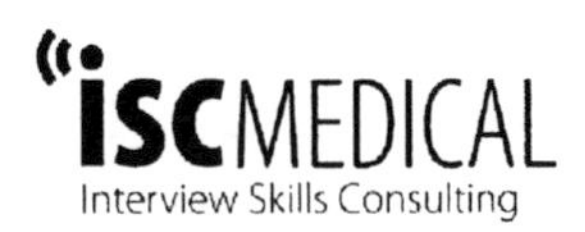

178	The following is true regarding hormonal changes during pregnancy.	OBS

a. Oestrogen levels rise, leading to an increase in breast and nipple size. True/False

b. Rising oestrogens lead to fluid retention. True/False

c. Prolactin rises only in the last trimester in preparation of delivery and postnatal feeding. True/False

d. Serum free cortisol rises during pregnancy. True/False

e. Progestogens increase body temperature. True/False

179	Regarding placenta previa.	OBS

a. If a low-lying placenta is identified, elective Caesarean section should be anticipated. True/False

b. A major placenta previa means that the placenta covers the internal os. True/False

c. Placenta previa is more common with velamentous insertion. True/False

d. Most units advocate early admission and monitoring prior to caesarean section of cases with major placenta previa. True/False

e. About 10% of early identified low lying placentas result in a placenta previa at term. True/False

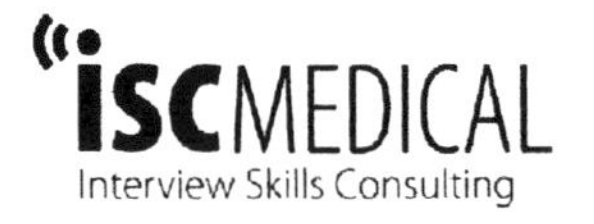

MCQs for GPVTS

OPHTHALMOLOGY

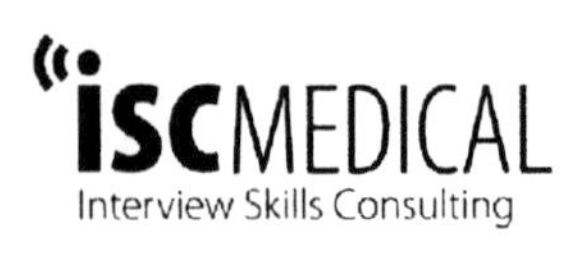

180 Pupils. **OPHTH**

a. The Argyll Robertson (AR) pupil is virtually pathognomic of neurosyphilis. True/False

b. A Marcus Gunn pupil will constrict if a bright enough light is shone in that eye. True/False

c. The Argyll Robertson (AR) pupil is often irregular in shape. True/False

d. The Holmes-Adie pupil is dilated in the resting state. True/False

e. The Holmes-Adie pupil does not react to light or accommodation. True/False

181 Myopia. **OPHTH**

a. Corrective lenses are convex. True/False

b. The globe is too long. True/False

c. Has been linked to an excess of close up work as a child. True/False

d. Retinal detachment is a recognised complication. True/False

e. Is associated with acromegaly. True/False

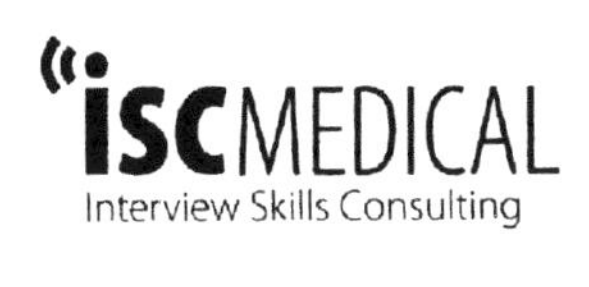

182 The following are features of anterior uveitis. **OPHTH**

a. Nystagmus. True/False

b. Pain on accommodation. True/False

c. Photophobia. True/False

d. Lacrimation. True/False

e. Small pupil. True/False

183 Keratitis. **OPHTH**

a. This is ulceration of the cornea. True/False

b. Typically a white spot may appear on the cornea. True/False

c. Dendritic ulcers are caused by herpes zoster virus. True/False

d. Fluorescein turns blue in corneal lesions. True/False

e. Virtually all cases are due to bacterial infections and chloramphenicol eye drops will suffice as treatment. True/False

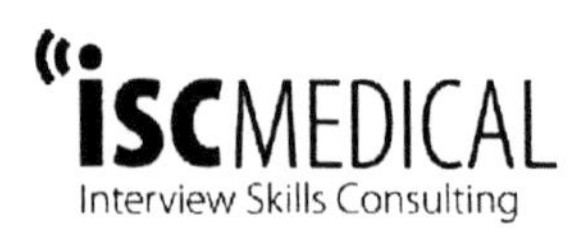

184 The following are features of acute closed angle glaucoma. **OPHTH**

a. Ectropion. True/False

b. Hypopyon. True/False

c. Vomiting. True/False

d. Dilated pupil. True/False

e. Cloudy cornea. True/False

185 Squints (Strabismus). **OPHTH**

a. With a convergent squint, the abnormal eye will move laterally when the normal eye is covered. True/False

b. Non-paralytic squints are often secondary to an underlying refractive error. True/False

c. Divergent squints are often intermittent. True/False

d. Many childhood squints will resolve spontaneously with visual stimuli and training techniques. If this fails, ophthalmology review may be of help. True/False

e. A pseudosquint can occur in Down's syndrome. True/False

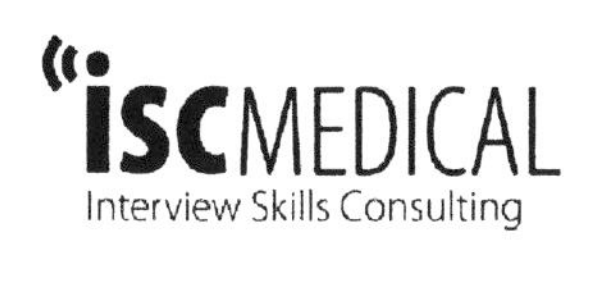

186 Retinoblastoma. **OPHTH**

a. Potentiation of the red reflex often occurs. True/False

b. Visual disturbance including blindness is most often the method in which this condition presents. True/False

c. Is associated with a significantly increased risk of bone and muscle tumours. True/False

d. Squint is a recognised feature. True/False

e. Often leads to proptosis. True/False

187 Superficial eye infections. **OPHTH**

a. Orbital cellulitis often involves anaerobic bacteria trapped in the lacrimal ducts. True/False

b. Orbital cellulitis is often bilateral due to autoinnoculation via the nasal sinuses. True/False

c. Orbital cellulitis requires prompt CT evaluation. True/False

d. Herpes zoster involving the tip of the nose is highly suggestive of later eye and corneal involvement. True/False

e. Under <1% of cases of shingles affect the ophthalmic division of the trigeminal nerve i.e. causing ophthalmic shingles. True/False

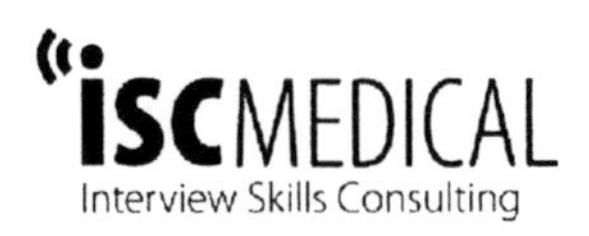

188 The following are recognised associations of dry eyes. **OPHTH**

a. Addison's disease. True/False

b. Old age. True/False

c. Lymphoma. True/False

d. Hypothyroidism. True/False

e. Psoriasis. True/False

189 Tears etc. **OPHTH**

a. The lacrimal gland is located on the lateral (temporal) aspect of the eye. True/False

b. An ectropion can lead to abnormal drainage of tears. True/False

c. Keratoconjunctivitis sicca is most commonly associated with an underlying rheumatological condition. True/False

d. Schober's test is used to evaluate abnormalities in tear volume. True/False

e. Pemphigoid can lead to abnormal formation of tears. True/False

190 Around the eye. **OPHTH**

a. Entropion is inturning of the eye lid. True/False

b. A stye is an inflammatory swelling of the eye lid. True/False

c. A pinguecula is a degenerative nodule on the cornea. True/False

d. A marginal cyst is a non-infected subtype of stye. True/False

e. A pterygium is a nodular growth on the eye lid that may require excision. True/False

191 Episcleritis. **OPHTH**

a. Tends to be painless. True/False

b. Is more superficial than scleritis. True/False

c. Virtually all cases are due to a connective tissue disorder. True/False

d. Is unlikely to case perforation of the globe. True/False

e. Acuity is usually not affected. True/False

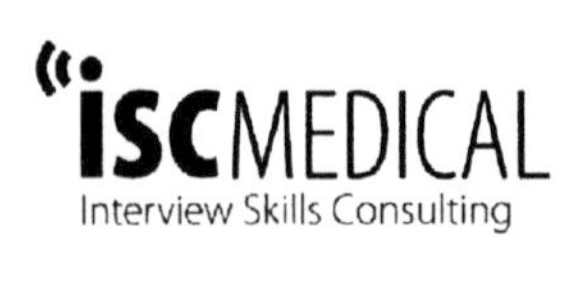

192 Treatments for glaucoma. **OPHTH**

a. Pilocarpine can lead to blurred vision. True/False

b. Timolol works by decreasing aqueous secretion. True/False

c. Timolol can induce bronchoconstriction. True/False

d. Flap-valve trabeculectomy can worsen the condition of cataracts. True/False

e. Latanoprost helps by decreasing flow of aqueous. True/False

193 Eye disease in the developing world. **OPHTH**

a. Keratomalacia is often accompanied by night blindness. True/False

b. Perforation of the cornea is a complication of keratomalacia. True/False

c. Vitamin A is given in pregnancy to prevent early onset of keratomalacia. True/False

d. Trachoma causes a follicular conjunctivitis. True/False

e. Trachoma is caused by Chlamydia trachomatis. True/False

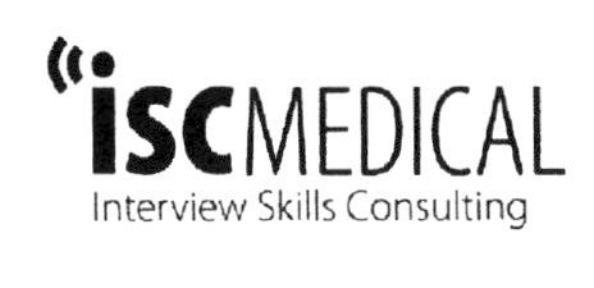

194 The following are recognised features of hypertensive retinopathy. **OPHTH**

a. Macular star. True/False

b. Angioid streaks. True/False

c. Hard exudates. True/False

d. Neovascularisation. True/False

e. Cotton wool spots. True/False

195 The following stages of diabetic retinopathy are correctly matched with the management strategy. **OPHTH**

a. Mild background retinopathy : non-urgent ophthalmology referral. True/False

b. Maculopathy : 6 monthly review and refer if and change in acuity. True/False

c. Preproliferative : non-urgent ophthalmology referral. True/False

d. Proliferative : urgent ophthalmology referral. True/False

e. Rubeosis : arrange assessment of visual fields and intraocular pressure. True/False

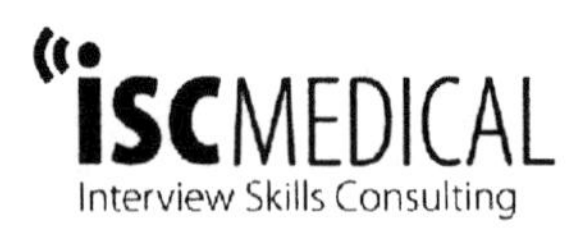

196 Diabetes and retinopathy. **OPHTH**

a. Type 1 diabetics tend to develop retinopathy within 5 years of diabetes diagnosis. True/False

b. Type 1 diabetics are more prone to maculopathy than type 2. True/False

c. Type 2 diabetics often have some degree of retinopathy at diagnosis of diabetes. True/False

d. Diabetes can exacerbate age-related macular degeneration. True/False

e. Blood pressure control has a substantial effect on diabetic retinopathy. True/False

197 The following are features of background diabetic retinopathy. **OPHTH**

a. Cotton wool spots. True/False

b. Venous beading. True/False

c. Blot haemorrhages. True/False

d. Microaneurysms. True/False

e. Hard exudates. True/False

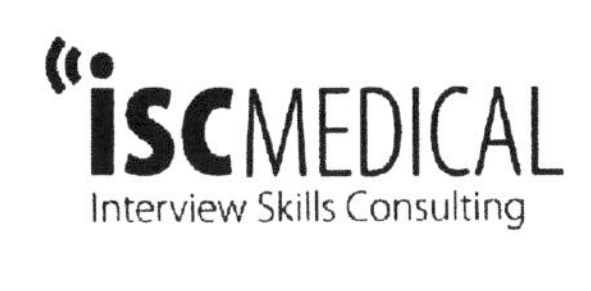

198 The following are recognised causes of retinal detachment. **OPHTH**

a. Intraocular melanoma. True/False

b. Retinitis pigmentosa. True/False

c. Branch retinal artery occlusion. True/False

d. Cataract surgery. True/False

e. Glaucoma. True/False

199 The following are recognised features of retinal detachment. **OPHTH**

a. Fortification spectra. True/False

b. Alteration to visual field. True/False

c. Haloes. True/False

d. Flashing lights. True/False

e. 'Floaters'. True/False

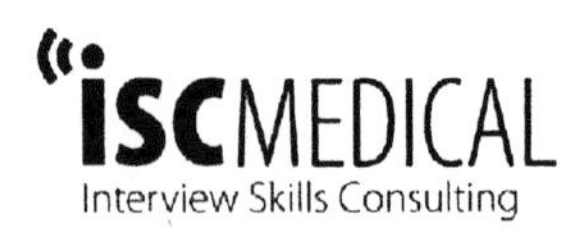

200 Eye drops. **OPHTH**

a. Tropicamide is a mydriatic. True/False

b. Miotics are used in glaucoma treatment. True/False

c. Eyes must always be screened for dendritic ulcers before steroid drops are used. True/False

d. Steroid drops can cause glaucoma. True/False

e. Fluorescein has anaesthetic properties. True/False

201 Cataracts. **OPHTH**

a. Can be treated in the early stages with pilocarpine which can decrease pressure effects on the lens. True/False

b. May present as a squint in children. True/False

c. Congenital cataracts tend to be localised on the lens. True/False

d. Up to a third of patients suffer posterior capsule opacification as a late complication from cataract surgery. True/False

e. After cataract surgery most patients will require a week of convalescence, before they can fully resume their activities. True/False

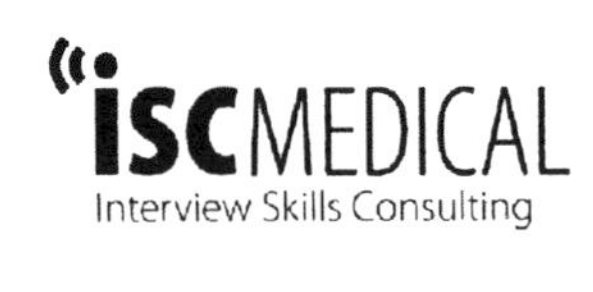

202 The following are common causes of choroidoretinitis. **OPHTH**

a. Cytomegalovirus. True/False

b. Toxoplasmosis. True/False

c. Herpes simplex virus. True/False

d. Varicella zoster virus. True/False

e. Mycobacterium tuberculosis. True/False

203 The following are recognised features of open angle glaucoma. **OPHTH**

a. Narrowing of the optic disc 'cup'. True/False

b. Arcuate scotoma. True/False

c. Gradual early loss of visual acuity. True/False

d. Raised intraocular pressure reducing arterial perfusion and causing disc pallor. True/False

e. Predominant nasal-superior visual field loss. True/False

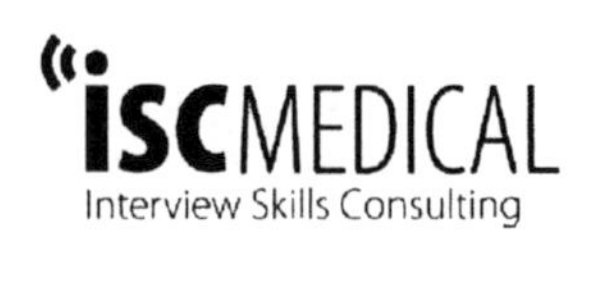

204 The following are recognised risk factors for developing glaucoma. **OPHTH**

a. Thyroid eye disease. True/False

b. Keratoconus. True/False

c. Diabetes mellitus. True/False

d. Afro-Caribbean ethnicity. True/False

e. Myopia. True/False

205 The following are recognised causes of optic atrophy. **OPHTH**

a. Syphilis. True/False

b. Hypocalcaemia. True/False

c. Friedrich's ataxia. True/False

d. Myotonic dystrophy. True/False

e. Alcohol abuse. True/False

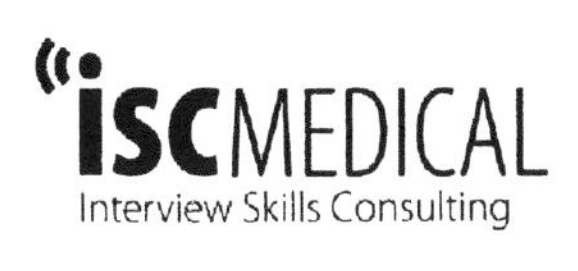

206	The following visual field defects are correctly matched to their possible cause.	OPHTH

a. Left superior quadrantanopia : Right parietal lobe lesion. True/False

b. Left horizontal hemianopia : Left optic nerve compression. True/False

c. Right homonymous scotoma : Lesion at tip of left occipital lobe. True/False

d. Arcuate scotoma : Glaucoma. True/False

e. Left homonymous hemianopia with macular sparing : Right optic tract lesion. True/False

207	Age related macular degeneration.	OPHTH

a. This is the most common cause of registrable blindness in the UK. True/False

b. The process is exacerbated by the toxic effects of tobacco. True/False

c. Drusen accumulation on the retina is a feature. True/False

d. Management involves photocoagulation of abnormal vessels near the fovea. True/False

e. A patient viewing gridlines as being distorted is a recognised feature. True/False

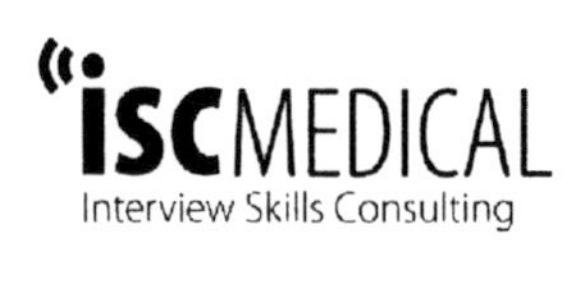

208 Sudden visual loss. **OPHTH**

a. When caused by vitreous haemorrhage, it often requires urgent removal by vitrectomy. True/False

b. If due to temporal or giant cell arteritis, visual loss is due to occlusion of the retinal arteries. True/False

c. In retinal artery occlusion, the retina is typically pale with a 'cherry red' dot at the macula. True/False

d. Is also caused by optic atrophy secondary to Paget's disease. True/False

e. Eye movements are painful with optic neuritis. True/False

209 Conjunctivitis. **OPHTH**

a. Follicular conjunctivitis is more often viral in aetiology. True/False

b. Acuity is often affected. True/False

c. Photophobia is often reported. True/False

d. Scratching and rubbing of the eye can lead to a subconjunctival haemorrhage which must be promptly referred in order to consider decompression. True/False

e. Sodium cromoglycate is a useful treatment for allergic conjunctivitis. True/False

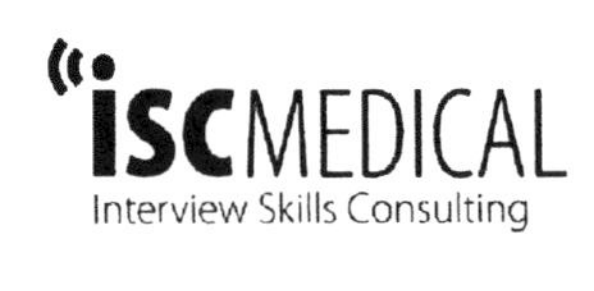

210 Ophthalmology terminology. **OPHTH**

a. Chemosis is drying of the conjunctiva. True/False

b. Keratomalacia is erosions on the cornea. True/False

c. Papillitis is inflammation of the optic nerve head. True/False

d. Anisocoria is distortion to the shape of the iris. True/False

e. A scotoma is a foreign body in the vitreous which can lead to visual disturbance, also known as a floater. True/False

211 The following are recognised causes of cataracts. **OPHTH**

a. Old age. True/False

b. Use of inhaled steroids. True/False

c. Sjögren's syndrome. True/False

d. Myotonic dystrophy. True/False

e. Vitiligo. True/False

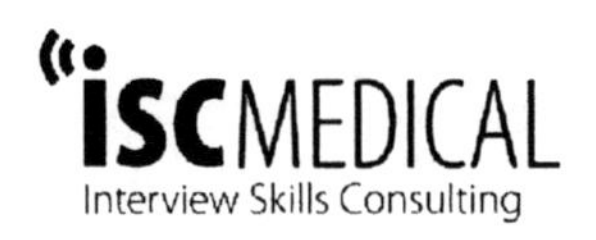
iSCMEDICAL
Interview Skills Consulting

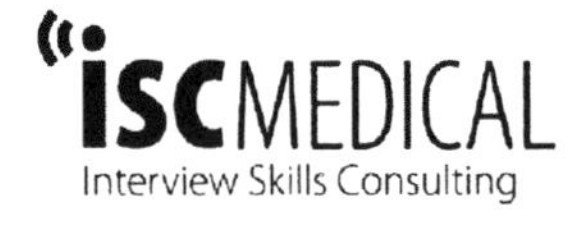

MCQs for GPVTS

ORTHOPAEDICS

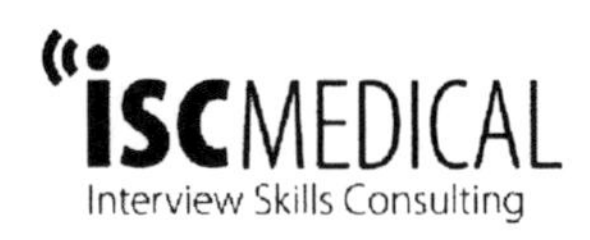

212 The following are recognised associations with Dupuytren's contracture. **ORTHO**

a. Anticonvulsant therapy. True/False

b. Peyronie's disease. True/False

c. Use of vibrating tools. True/False

d. Keyboard operators. True/False

e. Alcoholism. True/False

213 Neck and cervical spine problems. **ORTHO**

a. Persistent spasmodic torticollis is relieved by injections with botulinum toxin. True/False

b. Prolapsed cervical discs often affect levels C5 - C7. True/False

c. Wasting muscles in the hand may be the first sign of c-spine pathology. True/False

d. Cervical rib is a known risk factor for coarctation of the aorta. True/False

e. Cervical rib is known to cause impaired arterial supply to the arm. True/False

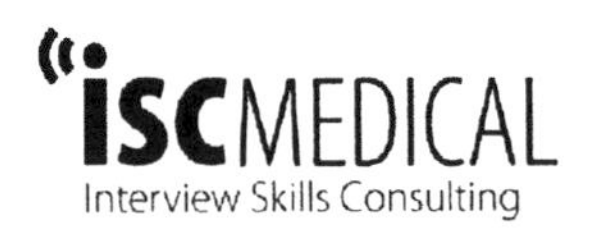

214 The shoulder joint. **ORTHO**

a. Recurrent dislocations often requires surgical repair. True/False

b. Atraumatic dislocations are mainly posterior. True/False

c. Traumatic dislocations are mainly anterior. True/False

d. Rotator cuff tears result in limited passive movement. True/False

e. Tears in supraspinatus are typified by loss of abduction up to 15 - 90 degrees. True/False

215 The following is true regarding the forearm and hand. **ORTHO**

a. Trigger finger is often due to a tendon nodule caused by osteoarthritis. True/False

b. Steroid injections are helpful in cases of trigger finger. True/False

c. Ganglia are swellings that connect with the joint capsule or tendon sheaths. True/False

d. If symptoms are purely cosmetic, ganglia are rarely treated by surgery. True/False

e. Tennis elbow (medial humeral epicondylitis) may be treated with steroid injections, but one must take care not to damage the ulnar nerve. True/False

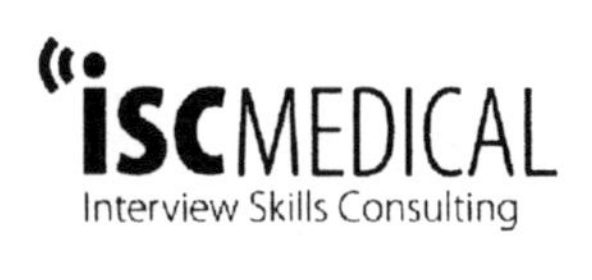

216 The following are recognised associations with scoliosis in the mediolateral plane. **ORTHO**

a. Poliomyelitis. True/False

b. Ankylosing spondylitis. True/False

c. Syringomyelia. True/False

d. Progressive deterioration in lung function requiring ventilatory support. True/False

e. Progressive oesophageal compression requiring stenting or assisted feeding. True/False

217 The following is true regarding Perthe's disease. **ORTHO**

a. It is virtually always unilateral. True/False

b. It can present with knee pain. True/False

c. It is rare beyond the age of 10 years. True/False

d. Steroid injection is effective in severe cases. True/False

e. Ultrasound is the investigation of choice. True/False

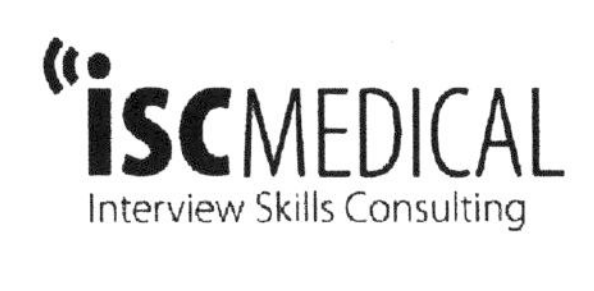

218 The following is true regarding slipped upper femoral epiphysis in children. **ORTHO**

a. It is uncommon before the age of 10. True/False

b. The significant majority of patients are obese. True/False

c. Most are bilateral. True/False

d. It is associated with delayed puberty. True/False

e. It is a risk factor for osteoarthritis in later life. True/False

219 The following are differential diagnoses for new-onset limp in a 6 year-old child. **ORTHO**

a. Perthe's disease. True/False

b. Osteogenesis imperfecta. True/False

c. Rickets. True/False

d. Tuberculosis. True/False

e. Talipes equinovarus. True/False

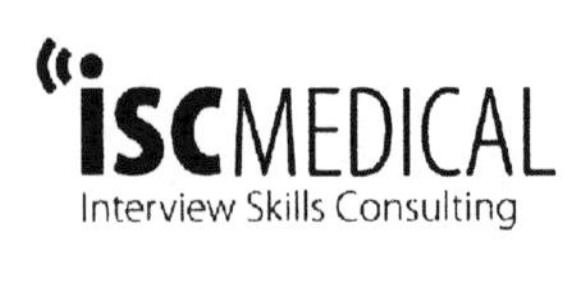

220 The following is true regarding 'DEXA scanning'. **ORTHO**

a. T score < -1 signifies osteoporosis. True/False

b. The T score signifies the number of standard deviations that someone's bone mineral density lies from the average bone mineral density for that person's age. True/False

c. The Z score signifies the number of standard deviations that someone's bone mineral density lies from the average bone mineral density for that person's gender and age. True/False

d. The risk of a pathological fracture doubles for every drop by 1 unit in T score. True/False

e. A T score > 0 is suggestive of Paget's disease. True/False

221 The following are recognised risks factors for development dysplasia of the hip. **ORTHO**

a. Breech birth. True/False

b. Maternal hypothyroidism. True/False

c. Di George's syndrome. True/False

d. Oligohydramnios. True/False

e. Prematurity. True/False

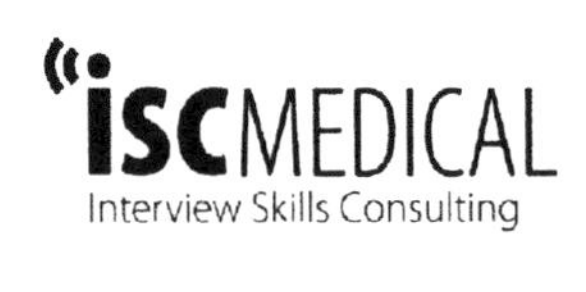

222 Problems with the knee joint. **ORTHO**

a. A knee joint swelling is most often due to an underlying connective tissue disease including rheumatoid or seronegative arthritis or due to an infection. True/False

b. A Baker's cyst is an inflammation of a bursa that can occur with rheumatoid arthritis. True/False

c. Osteochondritis dessicans is a cause of knee joint locking. True/False

d. A cruciate ligament tear is characterised by pain and tenderness especially along the joint line. True/False

e. Bursas may be treated with aspiration or steroid injection. True/False

223 Regarding the Salter and Harris classification of fractures. **ORTHO**

a. In type one, the fracture line follows the growth plate. True/False

b. Type one is the most common type of fracture. True/False

c. In type four, the fracture line crosses past the growth plate. True/False

d. Type six is also called a 'greenstick' fracture. True/False

e. Type five is a compression fracture. True/False

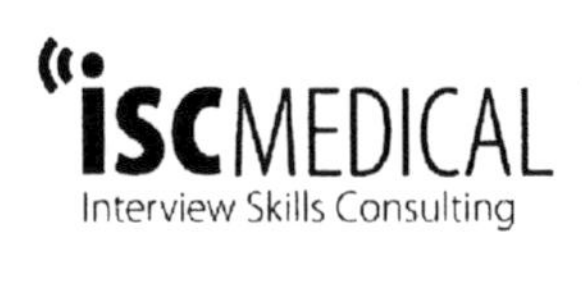

224	The following fractures are correctly matched with their definitions.	ORTHO

a. Colles' fracture : posterior angulation and displacement of the hand at the wrist. True/False

b. Smith's fracture : Volar angulation of distal radius fragment. True/False

c. Barton's fracture : Fracture of the ulnar styloid. True/False

d. Galeazzi : Fracture-dislocation of the carpometacarpal joint. True/False

e. Bennett's fracture : Fracture of shaft of radius. True/False

225	The following is true regarding Paget's disease.	ORTHO

a. May present with bilateral hearing loss. True/False

b. Skeletal changes typically lead to thoracic cage restriction and ventilatory failure. True/False

c. Is associated with increased osteoblastic activity. True/False

d. Alkaline phosphatase is used to monitor disease activity. True/False

e. Phosphate is often elevated. True/False

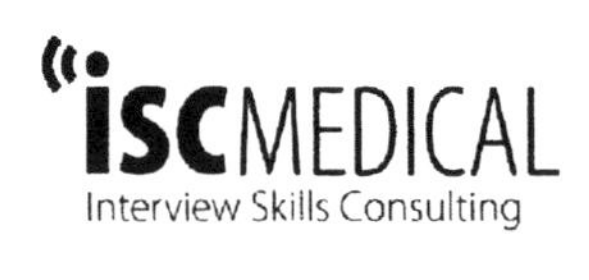

226 The following are recognised methods used to assess for osteopenia and osteoporosis. **ORTHO**

a. Quantitative computed tomography at the spine. True/False

b. Magnetic resonance imaging of the pelvis. True/False

c. Ultrasound measures at the heel. True/False

d. Doppler ultrasound at the wrist. True/False

e. Peripheral dual energy x-ray absorptiometry of the finger. True/False

227 The following is true regarding developmental dysplasia of the hip. **ORTHO**

a. The significant majority of cases are detected at the first neonatal check. True/False

b. A positive Ortolani test produces a dislocation relocation click as the femoral head returns to the acetabulum. True/False

c. Pelvic X-ray is the most useful imaging modality. True/False

d. Less than 20% of affected infants are male True/False

e. Hip abduction in frames or splints risks avascular necrosis of the femoral head. True/False

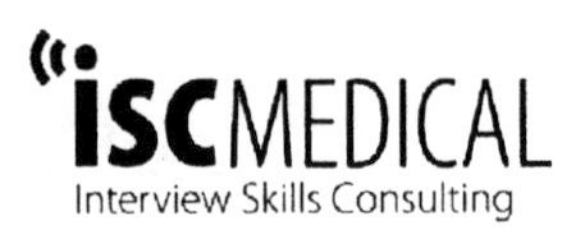

228 The following is true regarding adhesive capsulitis. **ORTHO**

a. The shoulder is painful at rest and tender if bearing weight in bed. True/False

b. This also known as frozen shoulder. True/False

c. Presentation may often follow minor injury to the shoulder. True/False

d. Active but not passive movement is reduced. True/False

e. Resolution of symptoms takes at most a few months. True/False

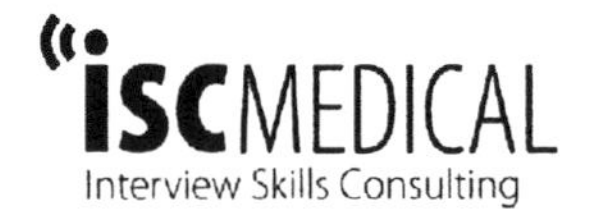

MCQs for GPVTS

PAEDIATRICS

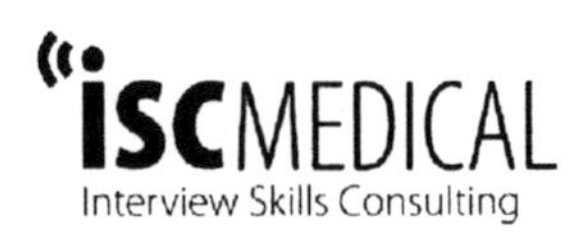

229 The following are recognised features of foetal hydrops. **PAEDS**

a. When ventilating the baby, high inspiratory pressures are required. True/False

b. Hypernatraemia. True/False

c. Hypoalbuminaemia. True/False

d. Hypertension. True/False

e. Pleural effusions. True/False

230 Respiratory distress syndrome. **PAEDS**

a. Air bronchograms are seen on chest X–ray. True/False

b. The severity is greatest at 2-4 hours of age. True/False

c. Is associated with group B streptococcal infection. True/False

d. Is caused by aspiration of meconium. True/False

e. This diagnosis should be applied to pre-term infants only. True/False

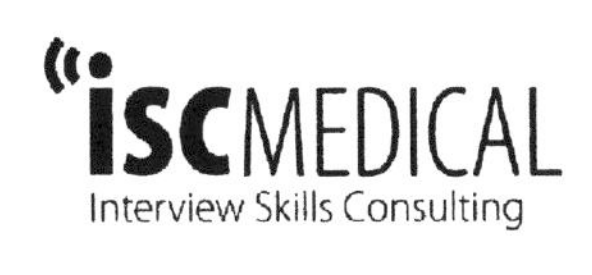

231 The following deliveries always necessitate the attendance of a paediatric team. **PAEDS**

a. Caesarean section. True/False

b. Twin birth. True/False

c. Ventouse delivery. True/False

d. Breech birth. True/False

e. Low lying placenta. True/False

232 Acute problems in a neonate. **PAEDS**

a. Sepsis often leads to severe acidosis and so bicarbonate is frequently required. True/False

b. Infection with staphylococcus epidermidis is often a problem. True/False

c. Creactive protein is a reliable marker of sepsis. True/False

d. Benzodiazepines are contraindicated for neonatal seizures. True/False

e. Hypomagnesaemia should be actively excluded in neonatal seizures. True/False

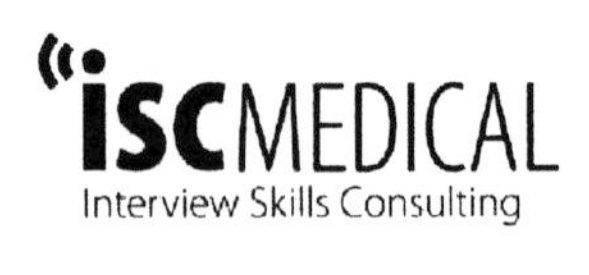

233 Neonatal jaundice. PAEDS

a. Within the first 24 hours it is often due to haemolysis. True/False

b. After day 5 it is most often abnormal and would warrant further investigation and treatment. True/False

c. Hypothyroidism is a cause of prolonged jaundice. True/False

d. If severe it may necessitate exchange blood transfusion. True/False

e. Biliary atresia presents from birth with pale stools and dark urine. True/False

234 Problems in a neonate. PAEDS

a. Nasogastric feeding is often used to prevent aspiration. True/False

b. Retinopathy of prematurity (RoP) is due to fragile retinal vessels being damaged after acute changes in blood pressure. True/False

c. Apnoeic attacks can be treated with caffeine. True/False

d. Intraventricular haemorrhage may be caused by hypoxia in a neonate. True/False

e. Intraventricular haemorrhage may be caused by hypercapnia in a neonate. True/False

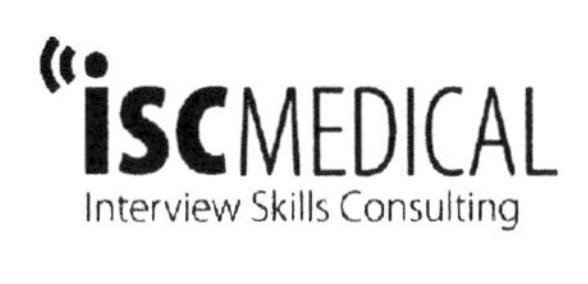

235 The following are abnormal if detected in the neonatal assessment. **PAEDS**

a. Head circumference 40cm. True/False

b. Single palmar crease. True/False

c. Mongolian spots on buttocks. True/False

d. Palpable liver edge. True/False

e. Per vaginal bleeding. True/False

236 The following are features of the Apgar scoring system. **PAEDS**

a. Heart rate. True/False

b. Oxygen saturation. True/False

c. Respiratory rate. True/False

d. Muscle tone. True/False

e. Reflex response to stimulation True/False

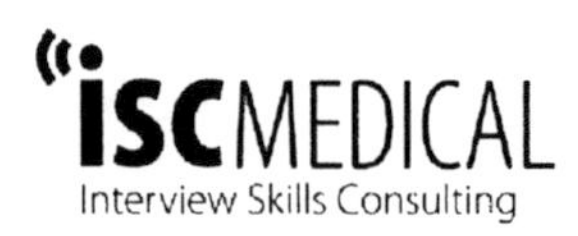

237 Murmurs. **PAEDS**

a. A thrill may just be a reflexion of turbulent flow secondary to tachycardia with fever or anxiety. True/False

b. A VSD murmur is best heard on the left side of the chest near the apex. True/False

c. Benign murmurs are heard in most children at some time in their early life. True/False

d. A Still's murmur is associated with juvenile Still's disease. True/False

e. A murmur from a PDA is a pansystolic murmur. True/False

238 Rhesus haemolytic disease. **PAEDS**

a. Only occurs in the second or subsequent pregnancies. True/False

b. Autoimmune haemolysis is a result of maternal IgD coating foetal red blood cells. True/False

c. Foetal blood sampling is contraindicated since this can precipitate haemolysis. True/False

d. The risk to the foetus of maternally derived antibodies is over once the baby is delivered. True/False

e. The presence of any Rhesus antibodies in the mother during pregnancy strongly suggests future haemolysis in the newborn. True/False

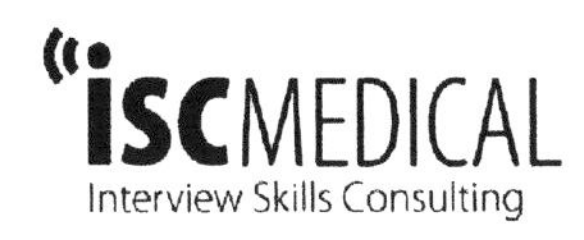

239 Specific types of epilepsy in a child. **PAEDS**

a. Reflex anoxic seizures are related to vagal hyperstimulation. True/False

b. If severe and recurrent, then anticonvulsants may be beneficial for reflex anoxic seizures. True/False

c. With infantile spasms, the child jerks then has unilateral usually facial twitching. True/False

d. Atonic epilepsy involves rapid loss of stance as the child is thrown to the ground. True/False

e. In rolandic epilepsy a child may suddenly throw themself to the floor. True/False

240 Spina bifida. **PAEDS**

a. The risk of spina bifida is increased in subsequent pregnancies if the woman has already had children with it. True/False

b. Hip dislocation is a recognised complication. True/False

c. The majority of patients will not be able to walk by late childhood even if they have done so at an earlier age. True/False

d. A woman being treated with phenytoin should take 400mcg folic acid per day preconceptually. True/False

e. Is a risk factor for multiple urinary tract infections and renal damage. True/False

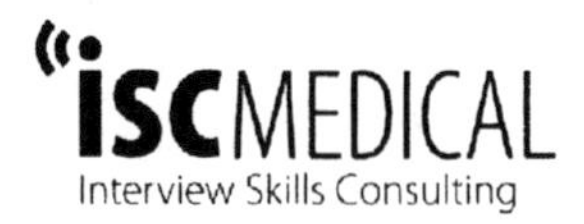

241 Conditions in the neonate. **PAEDS**

a. Neonates with necrotising enterocolitis should have all oral feeds stopped. True/False

b. Haemorrhagic disease of the newborn is due to a neonatal lack of vitamin K. True/False

c. Erythema toxicum are red macules, which often herald localised cellulitis. True/False

d. Red stains in a nappy are virtually always insignificant. True/False

e. Peeling skin is a common finding in postmature babies. True/False

242 The following signs are correctly matched with the degree of dehydration in a child. **PAEDS**

a. Decreased skin turgor : 5% dehydration. True/False

b. Dry mucous membranes : 5% dehydration. True/False

c. Sunken fontanelle : >10% dehydration. True/False

d. Drowsiness : 5% dehydration. True/False

e. Hypotension : >10% dehydration. True/False

243 Poisoning. PAEDS

a. Gastric lavage is of use in salicylate poisoning. True/False

b. Iron poisoning may lead to hypotension. True/False

c. Whole bowel irrigation has been used for iron poisoning. True/False

d. Gastric lavage or emetics are the best effective approach to petroleum poisoning. True/False

e. Hypoglycaemia is a common side effect of tricyclic antidepressant poisoning. True/False

244 Salicylate poisoning. PAEDS

a. Will give alkalosis in the early stages. True/False

b. N-acetylcysteine is the antidote of choice. True/False

c. A drug level is unreliable until at least 4 hours after estimated ingestion. True/False

d. Urinary alkalination is safe in children. True/False

e. Activated charcoal is contraindicated in most children. True/False

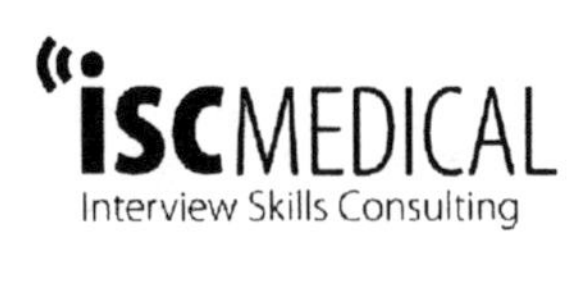

245 Signs of early acute raised intracranial pressure in a child include: **PAEDS**

a. Vomiting. True/False

b. Kussmaul's breathing. True/False

c. Papilloedema. True/False

d. Myoclonus. True/False

e. Diplopia. True/False

246 Brain tumours. **PAEDS**

a. Most tumours give generalised signs and specific cranial nerve lesions are rare. True/False

b. Cerebral tumours tend to cause seizures. True/False

c. Meningiomas are more common than gliomas. True/False

d. The majority of tumours arise from the posterior fossa. True/False

e. Medulloblastomas (cerebellar tumours) respond well to radiotherapy. True/False

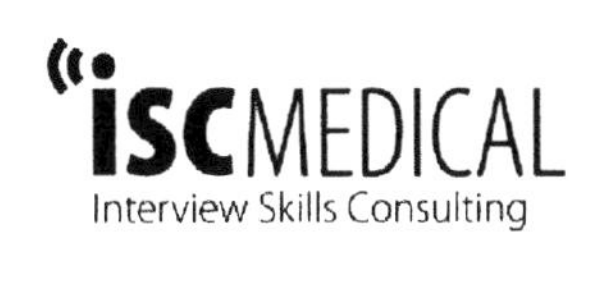

247 Meningitis. **PAEDS**

a. May present with poor feeding alone. True/False

b. The fontanelle is often depressed. True/False

c. Brudzinski's sign is neck pain and stiffness on hip flexion. True/False

d. Meningism and purpuric rash suggests meningitis and a lumbar puncture is indicated. True/False

e. A rash that blanches makes meningicoccus unlikely. True/False

248 The second heart sound (S2). **PAEDS**

a. Is normally split during inspiration. True/False

b. Is continually split throughout respiration with a PDA. True/False

c. The first part is the aortic valve closure followed by the pulmonary. True/False

d. There is no splitting with tetralogy of Fallot. True/False

e. The second part of S2 is louder in pulmonary hypertension. True/False

249 Febrile convulsions. PAEDS

a. Typical febrile convulsions can be partial or generalised but are always complex. True/False

b. Management involves educating parents and even giving them rectal benzodiazepines for use at home. True/False

c. Seizures are a risk after subsequent vaccinations. True/False

d. About 1% of children with febrile convulsions will go on to develop epilepsy. True/False

e. Is most commonly due to a transient infection (even viral) of the central nervous system. True/False

250 Childhood development. PAEDS

a. A baby is expected to hold its head steady by 4 months of age. True/False

b. Meaningful words put together in couplets are expected by 18 months. True/False

c. Almost all babies can walk by the age of 12 months. True/False

d. An infant is not expected to be able to transfer objects from hand to hand until a year of age. True/False

e. A baby is not expected to weight bear until 10 months. True/False

251 Management of epilepsy. **PAEDS**

a. Diazepam is the first drug of choice in status epilepticus. True/False

b. Carbamazepine is the drug of choice for absences. True/False

c. Vigabatrin levels must be measured from time to time. True/False

d. Lamotrigine is contraindicated in children. True/False

e. Carbamazepine is the best drug for use with infantile spasms. True/False

252 The following are recognised causes of abdominal distension in a child. **PAEDS**

a. Malabsorption. True/False

b. Urinary tract infection. True/False

c. Air swallowing. True/False

d. Pancreatic cysts. True/False

e. Gastro-oesophageal reflux disease. True/False

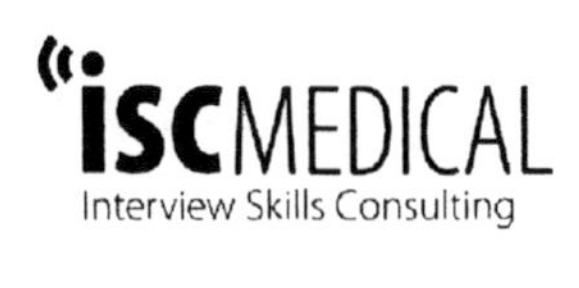

253 Diabetic ketoacidosis in a child. **PAEDS**

a. White cell count can rise even in the absence of infection. True/False

b. Cerebral oedema is a risk which is more apparent once fluid resuscitation has commenced. True/False

c. Patients may suffer from hypo or hypernatraemia. True/False

d. Can have features and tests suggestive of acute pancreatitis. True/False

e. Ketonuria and acidosis does not always mean ketoacidosis. True/False

254 Attention deficit disorder. **PAEDS**

a. Increased amount of speech and interrupting others are noted features. True/False

b. Can continue into early adulthood in some. True/False

c. Significant EEG abnormalities are a common finding. True/False

d. Maternal prenatal cannabis use is a noted risk factor. True/False

e. Is associated with familial learning disabilities. True/False

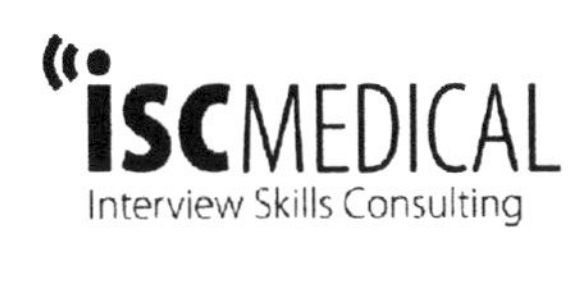

255 Genital anomalies and intersex. **PAEDS**

a. Testicular feminisation or androgen insensitivity syndrome leads to genetic males appearing as phenotypic females. Salt wasting from birth is a common and serious feature. True/False

b. Hypospadias should be treated with circumcision. True/False

c. The presence of a Barr body on buccal smear suggests female genotype. True/False

d. In congenital adrenal hyperplasia, there is reduced peripheral testosterone production and so a lack of a negative feedback to the adrenal gland, resulting in hyperplasia and increased adrenal androgen production. True/False

e. Aromatase deficiency leads to a lack of oestrogen in the body and, in males, can result in osteoporosis. True/False

256 The following meningitic organisms are correctly matched with the age groups of children which they typically affect. **PAEDS**

a. Listeria monocytogenes : infant. True/False

b. N. meningitidis : over 4 years. True/False

c. Pneumococcus : any age. True/False

d. E. coli : neonate. True/False

e. H. Influenzae : any age. True/False

257 The following is true of varicella zoster virus (VZV). **PAEDS**

a. Rash starts on the face. True/False

b. Acyclovir is contraindicated in those under 12. True/False

c. Maternal shingles during pregnancy does not lead to congenital VZV infection. True/False

d. Infection during pregnancy requires acyclovir treatment to the mother. True/False

e. It is particularly problematic in those with cystic fibrosis. True/False

258 Childhood viral exanthems. **PAEDS**

a. Roseola infantum is also known as slapped cheek virus. True/False

b. Roseola infantum is a human herpes virus (type 6). True/False

c. Roseola infantum gives a false positive Monospot ® test. True/False

d. Parvovirus B19 can cause haemolysis in those with thalassaemia. True/False

e. Parvovirus is a threat to pregnancy as it can cause foetal loss and hydrops fetalis. True/False

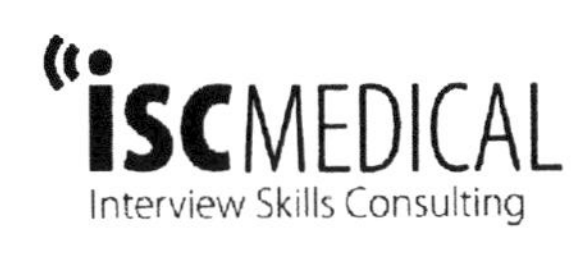

259 Mumps. **PAEDS**

a. The swollen parotid is typically painless. True/False

b. Patients are infective until the parotid swelling begins to decline. True/False

c. Deafness is a recognised complication. True/False

d. Pancreatitis is a recognised complication. True/False

e. Uveitis is a recognised complication. True/False

260 Measles. **PAEDS**

a. Koplik spots tend to fade before day 6. True/False

b. Rash starts on the trunk and spreads to cover the whole body. True/False

c. Patients are infective once Koplik spots develop. True/False

d. Secondary bacterial infections such as otitis are a frequent problem. True/False

e. Identified cases benefit from prophylactic antibiotics. True/False

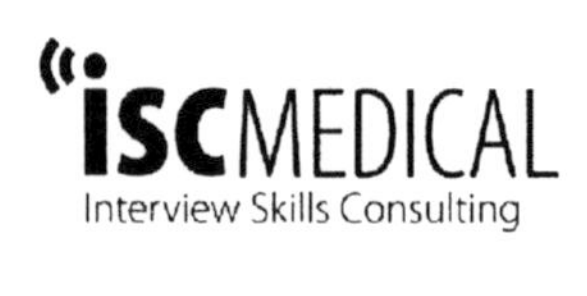

261 The following are recognised complications of Down's syndrome. **PAEDS**

a. Duodenal atresia. True/False

b. Pyloric stenosis. True/False

c. Nasal polyps. True/False

d. Coarctation of the aorta. True/False

e. Atrial septal defect. True/False

262 The following features aid recognition of Down's syndrome at birth. **PAEDS**

a. Hypotonia. True/False

b. High arched palate. True/False

c. Low IQ. True/False

d. Flat facial profile. True/False

e. Single palmar crease. True/False

263 The following conditions are usually screened for by gene probe techniques. **PAEDS**

a. Huntington's chorea. True/False

b. Edward's syndrome. True/False

c. Cystic fibrosis. True/False

d. Polycystic kidney disease. True/False

e. Phenylketonuria. True/False

264 Genetic terminology. **PAEDS**

a. Aneuploidy : Abnormal number of sex chromosomes. True/False

b. Nondisjunction of chromosomes : When at meiosis, one gamete gains more than one copy of a chromosome or chromosomes, and the other gamete loses a copy of that chromosome or chromosomes. True/False

c. Mosaicism : When an embryo is formed from more than one zygote (fertilised egg), so making a patchwork based on different genetic materials. True/False

d. Trisomy : Having three copies of a chromosome. True/False

e. Translocation : Where more than one chromosomes exchange genetic material between each other. True/False

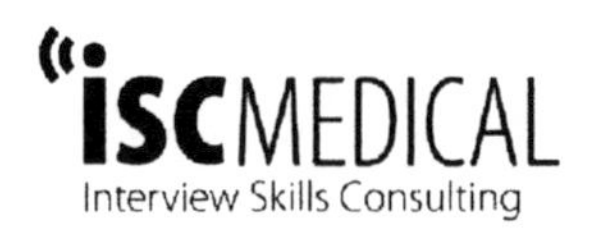

265 The following are recognised features of cerebral palsy. **PAEDS**

a. Hypotonia. True/False

b. Limb spasticity. True/False

c. Psychosis. True/False

d. Seizures. True/False

e. Adduction at the hip. True/False

266 The following are absolute contraindications to the 'MMR' vaccine. **PAEDS**

a. Prednisolone 5mg/day for a week 2 months ago. True/False

b. BCG vaccine taken 1 month ago. True/False

c. HIV. True/False

d. Allergy to egg. True/False

e. Spina bifida. True/False

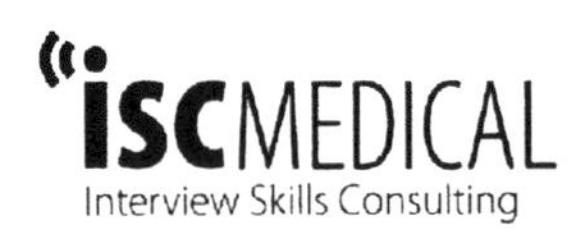

267 Management of congenital heart defects. PAEDS

a. In neonates, defects operate in a low pressure system and so endocarditis is rare. True/False

b. Digoxin may be used in a neonate in cardiac failure. True/False

c. Prostaglandin E1 is used to keep the ductus arteriosus open. True/False

d. Open heart surgery is the only option for pulmonary stenosis. True/False

e. Prenatal, intrauterine cardiac surgery is a possibility. True/False

268 Behavioural disorders. PAEDS

a. Pica is eating objects that aren't food, this is rarely normal and suggests an emotional disorder. True/False

b. Virtually all constipation is as a result of poor diet. True/False

c. Pharmaceutical therapy for enuresis is dangerous and so is rarely indicated. True/False

d. Enuresis can improve with alarm systems designed to sense a wet bed. True/False

e. School refusal is associated with parental depression and anxiety. True/False

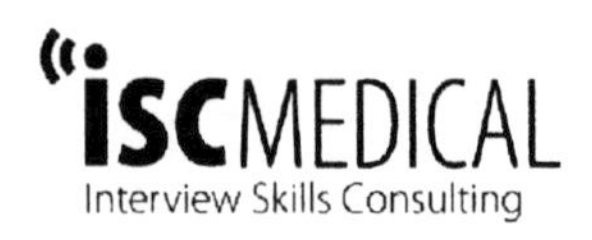

269 The following are recognised complications of chicken pox. **PAEDS**

a. Guillain - Barré syndrome. True/False

b. Pneumonia. True/False

c. Pancreatitis. True/False

d. Orchitis. True/False

e. Nephritis. True/False

270 Regarding cerebral palsy. **PAEDS**

a. Boys are affected more than girls. True/False

b. Most cases are due to birth trauma. True/False

c. Maternal alcohol consumption during pregnancy is implicated in some cases. True/False

d. Maternal herpes simplex acquisition during pregnancy has been implicated. True/False

e. Orthoxes are used to prevent flexion deformities. True/False

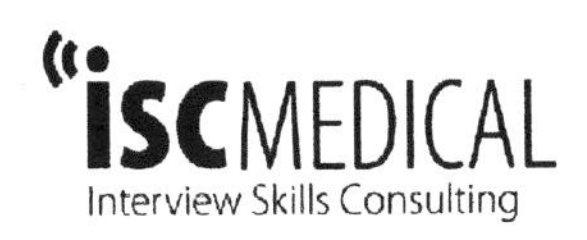

271 Iron deficiency anaemia in children.	PAEDS
a. Is now rare even in Caucasian children.	True/False
b. Is a feature of Meckel's diverticulum.	True/False
c. Is a feature of thalassaemia.	True/False
d. Is treated with ferrous sulphate orally.	True/False
e. Is a feature of coeliac disease.	True/False

272 Primary hypogammaglobulinaemia.	PAEDS
a. Is treated with infusions of immunoglobulin during acute infections.	True/False
b. Most cases present in infancy.	True/False
c. Can present with a syndrome similar to cystic fibrosis.	True/False
d. Is a cause of anaemia.	True/False
e. Seizures are a feature.	True/False

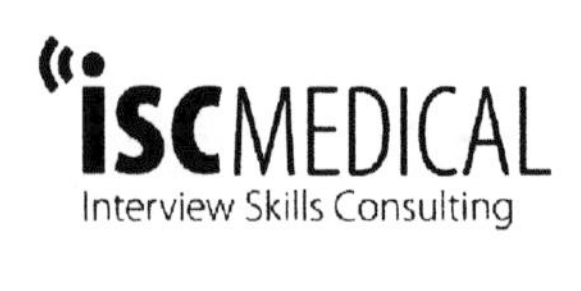

273 Recognised causes of precocious puberty include: **PAEDS**

a. Craniopharyngioma. True/False

b. Hypothyroidism. True/False

c. Tuberous sclerosis. True/False

d. Post meningitis. True/False

e. Mischievous child consuming mother's oral contraceptive pill. True/False

274 Precocious puberty. **PAEDS**

a. Is onset of puberty before the age of 10 in girls or 11 in boys. True/False

b. Can lead to short stature. True/False

c. Is treated with analogues of gonadotrophin releasing hormone GnRH. True/False

d. Can lead to electrolyte imbalance and salt wasting. True/False

e. Treatment does not reverse adrenal androgen secretion. True/False

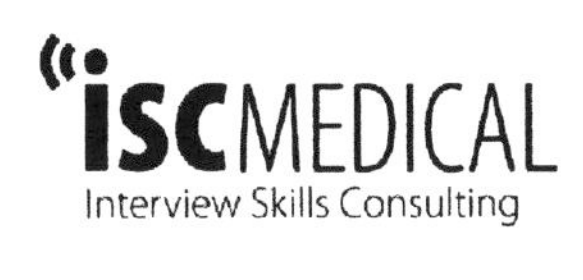

275 The following are recognised causes of intellectual impairment in a child. **PAEDS**

a. Lead poisoning. True/False

b. Marfan's syndrome. True/False

c. Coeliac disease. True/False

d. Kawasaki disease. True/False

e. Cystic fibrosis. True/False

276 The following are causes of congenital cyanotic heart disease. **PAEDS**

a. Pulmonary stenosis. True/False

b. Tetralogy of Fallot. True/False

c. Transposition of the great arteries. True/False

d. Total anomalous venous drainage. True/False

e. Hypoplastic left heart. True/False

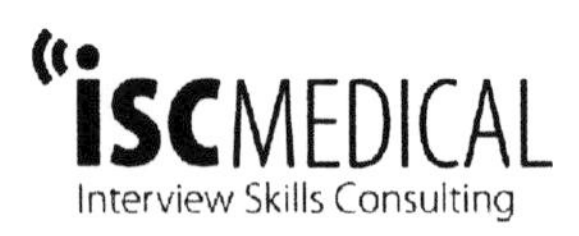

277 Signs in congenital heart disease. **PAEDS**

a. PDA gives a collapsing pulse. True/False

b. Coarctation presents from birth with poor peripheral pulses and shock. True/False

c. VSD gives a widely fixed split second heart sound and midsystolic murmur. True/False

d. ASD gives a harsh pansystolic murmur and thrill. True/False

e. Rib notching occur with a PDA due to high pressure flow in the pulmonary system. True/False

278 Immunisation schedule. **PAEDS**

a. Haemophilus influenzae type b (Hib) is given with MMR at 12-18months and 4-5 years. True/False

b. Diphtheria is given at 12 to 18 months then at 4 to 5 years. True/False

c. Polio is given at 2, 3 and 4 months then a booster between 4 and 5 years followed by a booster between 15 and 18 years. True/False

d. Pertussis is given at 2, 3 and 4 months only. True/False

e. Meningitis C (MC) vaccine is now given at 2, 3 and 4 months and a booster at 15 to 18 years. True/False

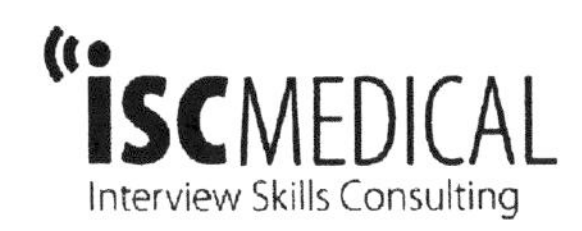

279	Vomiting in an infant.	PAEDS

a. Effortless vomiting is suggestive of pyloric stenosis. True/False

b. Bilious vomit is suggestive of duodenal obstruction. True/False

c. Two small vomits per day need not be investigated. True/False

d. Milk regurgitation during feeding is very common. True/False

e. Projectile vomiting occurs when lumps (projectiles) are detected in the vomit. True/False

280	The following are recognised complications of Cystic Fibrosis.	PAEDS

a. Steatorrhoea. True/False

b. Gallstones. True/False

c. Bowel obstruction. True/False

d. Nasal polyps. True/False

e. Male infertility. True/False

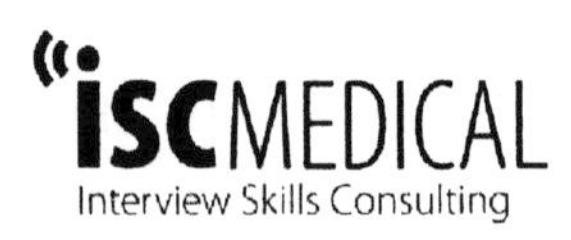

281 Urinary tract infection (UTI) in childhood. PAEDS

a. A micturating cystogram will assess for reflux uropathy. True/False

b. The majority of cases have an underlying anatomical abnormality. True/False

c. Is more common in circumcised boys than non circumcised. True/False

d. Ultrasound scanning is a useful method to exclude scarring from reflux nephropathy. True/False

e. With good aseptic technique, any organisms found from a suprapubic aspirate are highly suggestive of UTI. True/False

282 Diarrhoea in childhood. PAEDS

a. Temporary lactose intolerance may follow gastroenteritis. True/False

b. Toddler diarrhoea is usually due to a viral enteritis. True/False

c. Bloody diarrhoea is commonly due to inflammatory bowel disease. True/False

d. Green stools are common in those feeding on cow's milk. True/False

e. If a parent observes liquid stools for more than a week in an infant, they should seek a medical opinion. True/False

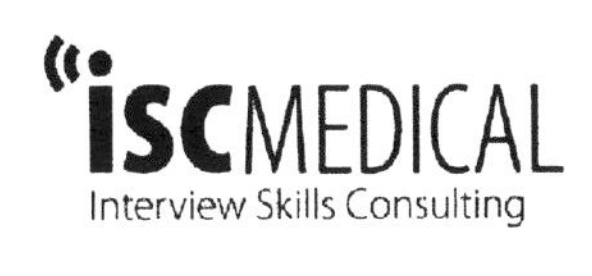

283 Malnutrition in a child. **PAEDS**

a. Marasmus is protein deficiency. True/False

b. Protein and mineral replacement must be swift to prevent irreversible damage from deficiency. True/False

c. Is known to lead to skin depigmentation. True/False

d. Can cause diarrhoea. True/False

e. Parenteral feeding is required to avert those at risk of renal failure. True/False

284 The following are recognised causes of short stature. **PAEDS**

a. Psychological abuse. True/False

b. Thyrotoxicosis. True/False

c. Cystic Fibrosis. True/False

d. Homocystinuria. True/False

e. Lead poisoning. True/False

285 Coeliac disease. **PAEDS**

a. Children almost always remain gluten intolerant for life. True/False

b. Rice and maize are not tolerated. True/False

c. Is associated with non-insulin dependent diabetes mellitus. True/False

d. Anti-endomysial antibodies are a useful test. True/False

e. Is associated with anaemia. True/False

286 The following is true of cystic fibrosis. **PAEDS**

a. A sweat test may be falsely positive in a patient with eczema. True/False

b. Presence or absence of the delta F 508 gene mutation can confirm or exclude the diagnosis. True/False

c. Most children are chronically infected with Pseudomonas aeruginosa. True/False

d. Supplementation of fat soluble vitamins is commonplace. True/False

e. Nebulised antibiotics and mucolytics taken at home have been found to decrease the number of hospital admissions. True/False

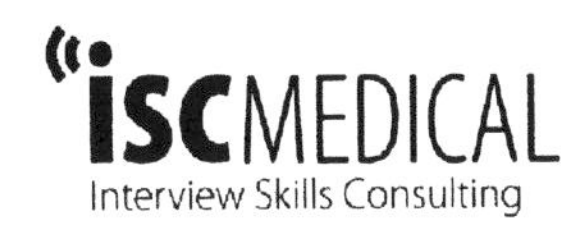

287 Nappy rash. **PAEDS**

a. Is often associated with a mycosis. True/False

b. Candidiasis is rare. True/False

c. Can resolve with more frequent nappy changes. True/False

d. Is commonly associated with an atopic reaction to toiletry products. True/False

e. Emollient creams are useful to aid resolution. True/False

288 The following are recognised risks for premature delivery. **PAEDS**

a. Pre-eclampsia. True/False

b. Short maternal stature. True/False

c. Tobacco smoking. True/False

d. Alcohol consumption. True/False

e. Multiple pregnancy. True/False

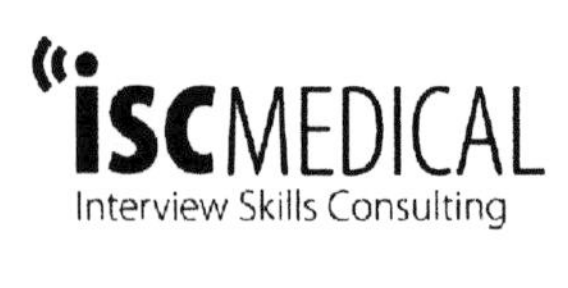

289 Crying in infancy. **PAEDS**

a. Can be reduced if a baby is fed by adult dictated intervals. True/False

b. Is associated with sudden infant death syndrome. True/False

c. Flexion of the baby's leg is suggestive of colic in a 3 month old baby. True/False

d. May be a sign of parental relationship difficulties. True/False

e. Screaming infers that a baby is in acute pain. True/False

290 The following is true regarding premature delivery. **PAEDS**

a. Babies delivered before 32 weeks have an increased risk of aspiration and should not be orally fed for several weeks. True/False

b. Up to 3 quarters of neonates born at 24 weeks do not survive. True/False

c. Delivery before 30 weeks is associated with subsequent learning difficulties. True/False

d. Most premature infants are also small for gestational age. True/False

e. Preterm infants have a greater risk of subsequent autoimmune conditions such as rheumatoid arthritis and diabetes mellitus. True/False

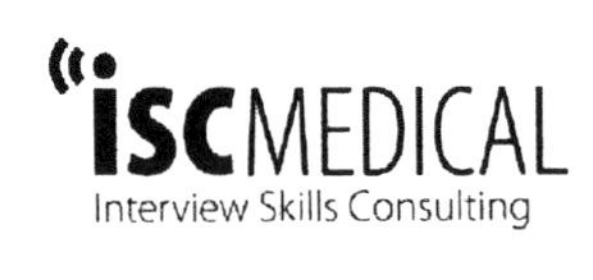

291 The following terms and definitions are correctly matched. **PAEDS**

a. Small for gestational age : neonate weighing 2000g delivered at 36 weeks. True/False

b. Preterm and low birth weight : neonate weighing 2600g delivered at 36 weeks. True/False

c. Low birth weight : neonate weighing < 2750g. True/False

d. Small for gestational age : Any preterm baby regardless of absolute weight. True/False

e. Preterm : Any baby delivered before 40 weeks gestation. True/False

292 Bottle Feeding. **PAEDS**

a. Bottle feed must be warmed. True/False

b. Follow-on milk contains a protein mix designed to delay gastric emptying and reduce hunger. True/False

c. Boiled water must be used. True/False

d. Inadequate reconstitution can lead to dangerous hypernatraemia. True/False

e. Soya milk is contraindicated in infants. True/False

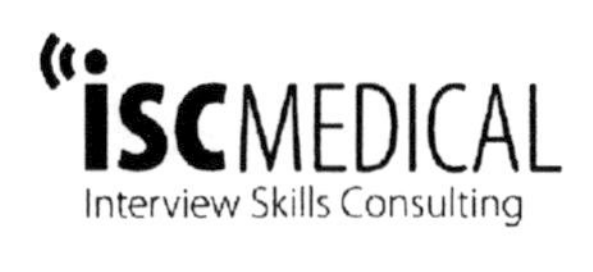

293 The following are benefits of breast feeding. **PAEDS**

a. Stimulates uterine contractions in the mother and so reduces rates of post partum haemorrhage. True/False

b. Reduces the later risk of rheumatoid arthritis in the recipient. True/False

c. Reduces the risks of infantile diarrhoea. True/False

d. Reduces the risk of later osteoporosis. True/False

e. Reduces the rate of later development of endometrial cancer in the mother. True/False

294 Henoch Schönlein purpura. **PAEDS**

a. Gastrointestinal bleeding is a noted complication. True/False

b. Children will require some form of immunosuppression even if it is just steroids alone. True/False

c. Purpura is over extensor surfaces. True/False

d. Renal disease is often in the form of nephrotic syndrome. True/False

e. Platelet count is reduced. True/False

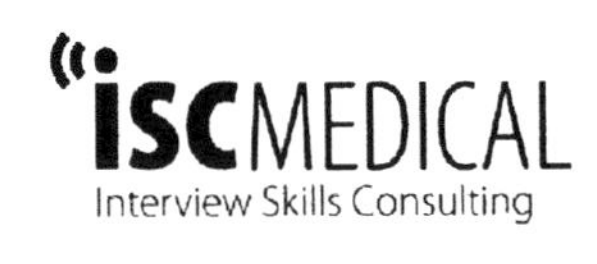

295 Cryptorchidism. **PAEDS**

a. Is associated with later testicular cancer. True/False

b. Is associated with later risk of torsion of testes. True/False

c. Is associated with later infertility. True/False

d. If testes are simply retractile, no surgery is required. True/False

e. Is commonly associated with hypospadias. True/False

296 Failure to thrive. **PAEDS**

a. In infancy, it describes poor weight gain. True/False

b. Almost all is due to undernutrition. True/False

c. Positive mid stream urine sample makes a urinary tract infection very likely. True/False

d. Up to the first 4 months, coeliac disease is not likely. True/False

e. Input from community visitors is useful in management. True/False

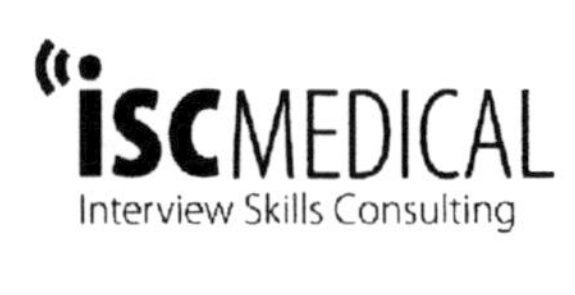

297 The following are true of phenylketonuria. **PAEDS**

a. It is routinely screened for prenatally. True/False

b. Dietary supplementation is part of management. True/False

c. May lead to phobic anxiety disorders. True/False

d. Is associated with deficits in attention. True/False

e. Is associated with demyelination. True/False

298 The following tasks/tests are correctly matched with their category within the Denver developmental screening test. **PAEDS**

a. Plays ball with examiner : Gross motor. True/False

b. Laughs : Language. True/False

c. Builds a tower of 8 cubes : Fine motor-adaptive. True/False

d. Gives first and last name : Personal-social. True/False

e. Does-up buttons on clothes : Fine motor-adaptive. True/False

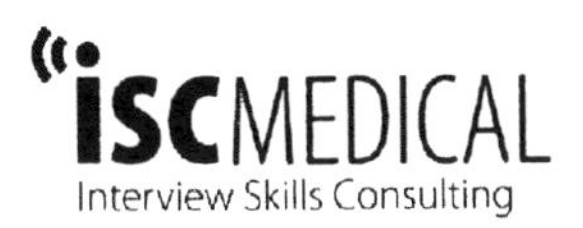

299 Sudden infant death syndrome (SIDS). **PAEDS**

a. This is the most common cause of death in infants over 1 week of age. True/False

b. Most cases end up being caused by smoke inhalation or other respiratory distress. True/False

c. Duvet bedding is discouraged and light blankets favoured in order to reduce the risk of SIDS. True/False

d. If the infant is a twin, the surviving twin should be admitted to hospital for investigations. True/False

e. Placing a baby on its back is intended to reduce risk by preventing obstruction to breathing. True/False

300 The following tasks from the Denver developmental test should be attainable by a child of the age stated. **PAEDS**

a. Kicks a football : 3 years old. True/False

b. Drinks from a cup : 16 months old. True/False

c. Copies a circle : 2 years old. True/False

d. Jumps up and down on spot : 18 months old. True/False

e. Feeds self a cracker : 8 months. True/False

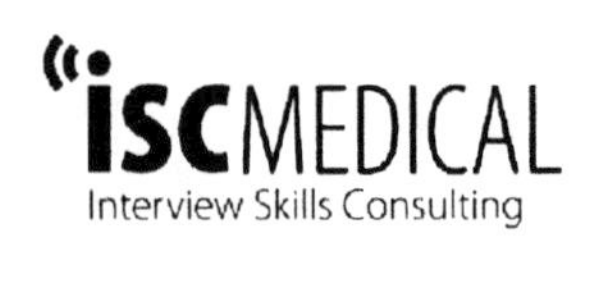

301	The following are recognised associations with hypothyroidism in childhood.	PAEDS

a. Prematurity. True/False

b. Hashimoto's thyroiditis. True/False

c. Neurofibromatosis. True/False

d. Down's syndrome. True/False

e. Tuberous sclerosis. True/False

302	The following is true regarding epiglottitis.	PAEDS

a. Fever is variable. True/False

b. Intubation is commonplace. True/False

c. Drooling is a frequent feature. True/False

d. The administration of antibiotics should be delayed until an airway is sited. True/False

e. Cough is prominent. True/False

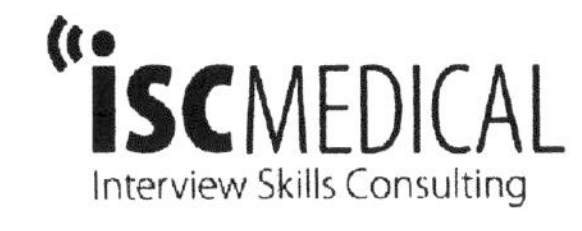

303 Acute bronchiolitis. **PAEDS**

a. Fever is typically high after a prodrome of coryza. True/False

b. Rates have reduced since the introduction of the 'Hib' vaccine. True/False

c. Steroids are of use in up to a third of cases. True/False

d. Is the most common lower respiratory infection in children. True/False

e. Antibiotics are generally not indicated. True/False

304 The following are recognised features of diphtheria. **PAEDS**

a. Tonsillitis. True/False

b. Nasal discharge. True/False

c. Cranial neuropathies. True/False

d. Myocarditis. True/False

e. Dysarthria. True/False

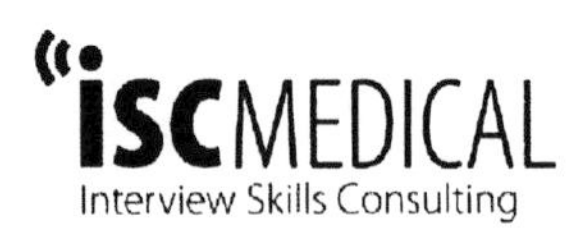

305 The following is true regarding viral croup. **PAEDS**

a. Onset is over a few days. True/False

b. Most cases are managed at home. True/False

c. Stridor is constant feature. True/False

d. Nebulised adrenaline is a treatment option. True/False

e. Drooling is a common feature. True/False

306 Whooping cough. **PAEDS**

a. Cough is worse at night. True/False

b. Pertusis antitoxin is an effective treatment. True/False

c. Diagnosis is aided by nasopharyngeal aspiration. True/False

d. Incubation period is 2-5 days. True/False

e. Violent coughing results in multiple petechiae and even intracranial haemorrhage. True/False

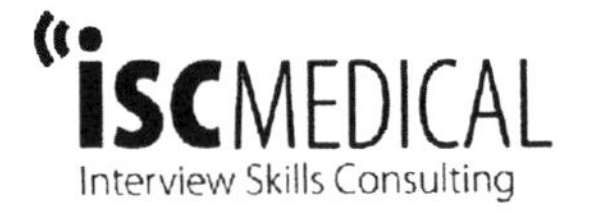

MCQs for GPVTS

PSYCHIATRY

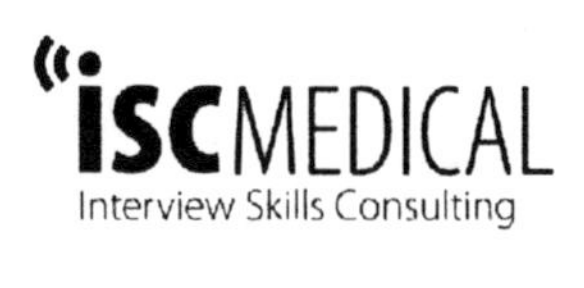

307 The following have been implicated in the aetiology of schizophrenia. **PSYCH**

a. Premature rupture of membranes before delivery. True/False

b. Diet poor in vitamin E. True/False

c. MMR vaccine. True/False

d. Autumn births True/False

e. Maternal alcohol consumption. True/False

308 The following is true regarding treatment of depression. **PSYCH**

a. Biological features of depression have been said to predict a good response to antidepressant drugs. True/False

b. Antidepressants are often not completely effective if a significant anxiety disorder is also present. True/False

c. Antipsychotics have a role. True/False

d. Antidepressants in those with bipolar disorder can precipitate a manic episode. True/False

e. Anhedonia with several other markers of depression for at least two weeks is an accepted guide to consider commencing antidepressant drugs. True/False

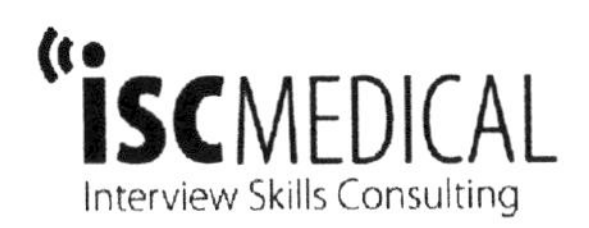

309 The following is true regarding depression. **PSYCH**

a. Hormones are of benefit in perimenopausal depression. True/False

b. The presence of hallucinations implies an underlying psychosis instead of depression. True/False

c. Electroconvulsive therapy is now very rarely performed and has been superceded by psychological and medical treatments. True/False

d. Prognosis is poorer when biological symptoms are present. True/False

e. St John's Wort (hypericum perforatum) is a safe alternative for those concerned about the side-effects of standard antidepressant treatments. True/False

310 The following are biological symptoms of depression. **PSYCH**

a. Waking early in the morning. True/False

b. Hyperphagia. True/False

c. Loss of libido. True/False

d. Poor eye contact. True/False

e. Urinary frequency. True/False

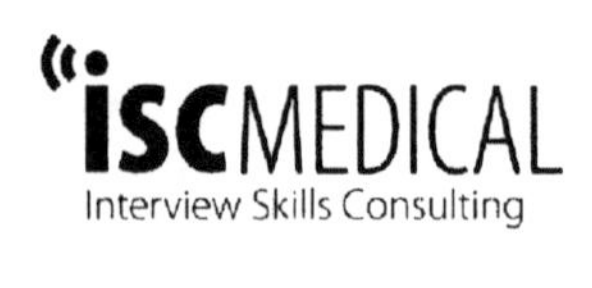

311	The following are features which form part of a list of criteria used to diagnose major depression.	PSYCH

a. Increased daytime tiredness. True/False

b. Insomnia. True/False

c. Inability to concentrate at work. True/False

d. Self blame. True/False

e. Amnesia. True/False

312	The following is true regarding postnatal depression.	PSYCH

a. Antidepressants have to cross the blood brain barrier and are therefore prone to enter breast milk. True/False

b. Postnatal depression not only affects the mother but has been shown to have a long term effect on social development of the child. True/False

c. Electroconvulsive therapy is a valuable treatment option. True/False

d. Oestrogen patches have been shown to be effective therapy. True/False

e. Suicide is the most common cause of maternal mortality. True/False

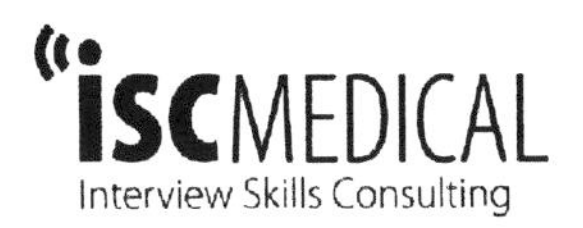

313 Which of the following terms are correctly defined? **PSYCH**

a. An auditory hallucination experienced at a time other than pre or just post sleep indicates a mental disorder. True/False

b. Tactile hallucinations tend to suggest an organic disorder. True/False

c. A pseudohallucination is where a stimulus is picked up, but is perceived differently to others. E.g. the sound of a car interpreted as the roar of pride of lions. True/False

d. A delusional perception is where someone thinks that they can sense something but they can't (e.g. when hearing a dog bark they believe they can hear the dog speak). True/False

e. An obsessional thought is a type of hallucination that is recurrent and obtrusive. True/False

314 The following are recognised features of bulimia nervosa. **PSYCH**

a. Pruritis. True/False

b. Haematemasis. True/False

c. Gastric rupture. True/False

d. Enlargement of parotid gland. True/False

e. Erosion to dental enamel. True/False

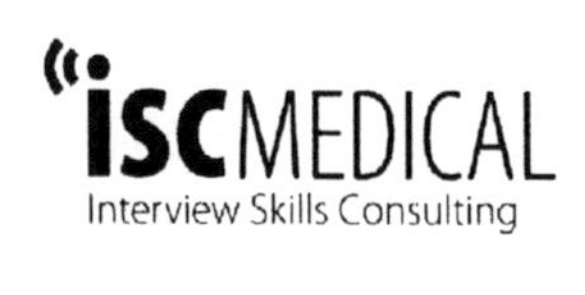

315 The following are recognised causes of dementia. **PSYCH**

a. Huntington's disease. True/False

b. Parkinson's disease. True/False

c. Multiple sclerosis. True/False

d. Schistosomiasis. True/False

e. HIV. True/False

316 The following are regarded as negative features of schizophrenia. **PSYCH**

a. Passivity of thought (thought insertion). True/False

b. Poor concentration. True/False

c. Blunted affect. True/False

d. Tardive dyskinesia. True/False

e. Social withdrawal. True/False

317 The following is true regarding delirium. **PSYCH**

a. It is a common feature for those with bipolar disorder experiencing manic episodes. True/False

b. Is often attributed to an underlying dementia. True/False

c. May often feature visual hallucinations. True/False

d. Features are often worse in the evenings. True/False

e. May be caused by a transient ischaemic attack. True/False

318 The following are essential components of a 'dementia screen' for an elderly patient with confusion. **PSYCH**

a. B12 and folate levels. True/False

b. Transferrin saturation. True/False

c. C reactive protein. True/False

d. Thyroid stimulating hormone. True/False

e. Plasma caeruloplasmin. True/False

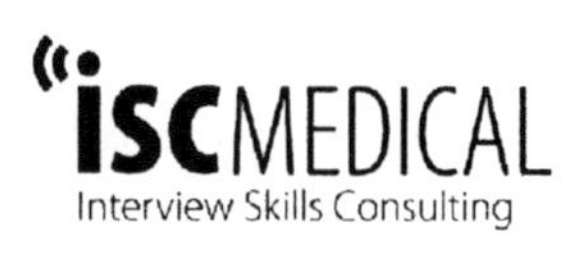

319 The following features make the diagnosis of depression more likely than dementia in cases of cognitive impairment. **PSYCH**

a. Varied response on repeated testing. True/False

b. The patient picks on their faults when given test results. True/False

c. The patient complains of poor memory. True/False

d. Memory loss is of recent events rather than global. True/False

e. The patient demonstrates apraxias. True/False

320 The following behaviours are correctly matched with the most likely affective state. **PSYCH**

a. Sitting on the edge of the seat : Mania. True/False

b. Poor eye contact : Anxiety. True/False

c. Slowness of thought : Depression. True/False

d. Expansive and theatrical gesticulations : Anxiety. True/False

e. Hips flexed and hugging ones knees : Depression. True/False

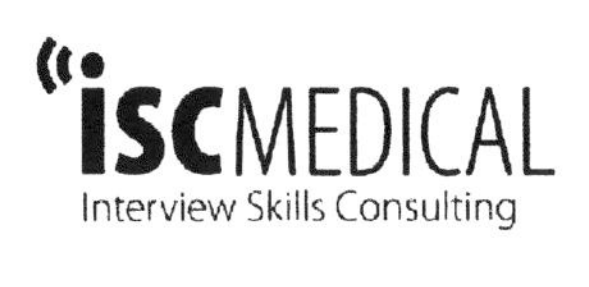

321 The following are recognised features of anxiety disorders. **PSYCH**

a. Irregular palpitations. True/False

b. Nausea. True/False

c. Lack of concentration. True/False

d. Increased libido. True/False

e. Tingling sensations. True/False

322 The following is true regarding bipolar affective disorder. **PSYCH**

a. Lithium remains the treatment of choice for many with bipolar disorder especially for rapid cyclers. True/False

b. Hypomania refers to euphoria without all the other features of mania. True/False

c. Cyclothymia means more than 4 episodes of either mania or depression in a year. True/False

d. Rapid cycling refers to changing out of one episode straight into another e.g. from mania straight into a period of depression with no period of normal mood in between. True/False

e. Switching refers to patients who flip between mania and depression within an episode of illness. True/False

323 The following are features of lithium overmedication. **PSYCH**

a. Tremors. True/False

b. Blurred vision. True/False

c. Polyuria. True/False

d. Hyperglycaemia. True/False

e. Accelerated hypertension. True/False

324 The following are recognised side effects of lithium therapy. **PSYCH**

a. SIADH. True/False

b. Alopecia. True/False

c. Constipation. True/False

d. Thyroid dysfunction. True/False

e. Renal tubular acidosis. True/False

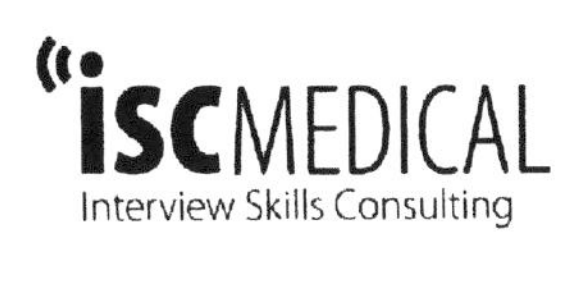

325 Suicide and self harm. **PSYCH**

a. Completed suicide is more common in males than females. True/False

b. Self harm is more common in males than females. True/False

c. Global suicide rates are slowly declining. True/False

d. Suicide is becoming more common in younger age groups. True/False

e. Many patients who complete suicide will have seen their GP with problems in a short period prior to the event. True/False

326 The following are recognised features or tests of the mental state examination. **PSYCH**

a. Asking someone to spell a word backwards. True/False

b. Noting whether someone wears make-up. True/False

c. Observing someone's posture. True/False

d. Asking someone to name 'the odd one out' from a list of numbers or nouns. True/False

e. Testing recall of a few objects or an address. True/False

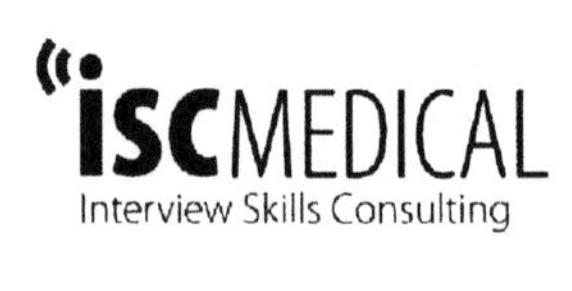

327 The following are 'first rank' symptoms of schizophrenia. **PSYCH**

a. Thought echo. True/False

b. Ideas of reference. True/False

c. Knight's move thinking. True/False

d. Thought broadcast. True/False

e. Passivity of actions (under control of an external force). True/False

328 Specific anxiety disorders. **PSYCH**

a. Panic disorder or panic attacks comprise paroxysms of intense anxiety often precipitated by a specific situational cue. True/False

b. "Modelling" is a cognitive behavioural technique used in the treatment of panic disorder. True/False

c. Phobic anxiety disorders tend not to be situational. True/False

d. Agoraphobia is a fear that being amongst people will lead to humiliation or embarrassment. True/False

e. Needing to escape and run away is a key feature of a panic attack. True/False

329 The following are recognised features of Wernicke's encephalopathy. **PSYCH**

a. Nystagmus. True/False

b. Confusion. True/False

c. Ataxia. True/False

d. Confabulation. True/False

e. Ophthalmoplegia. True/False

330 The following are features of alcohol dependence syndrome. **PSYCH**

a. Guilt associated with heavy drinking. True/False

b. A compulsion to drink alcohol. True/False

c. Tolerance to higher doses of alcohol. True/False

d. Anger towards others when told that drinking should be reduced. True/False

e. Withdrawal symptoms present after drinking stops. True/False

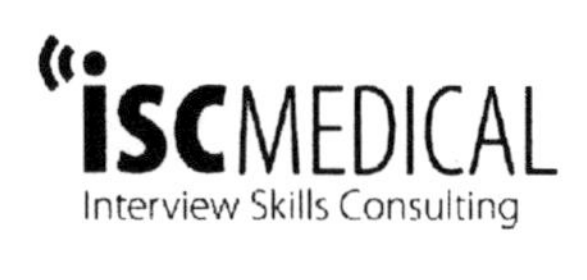

331 The following are recognised biochemical markers of neuroleptic malignant syndrome. **PSYCH**

a. Raised CRP. True/False

b. Raised CPK. True/False

c. Raised ESR. True/False

d. Raised WCC. True/False

e. Raised LDH. True/False

332 The following are recognised clinical features of neuroleptic malignant syndrome. **PSYCH**

a. Tonic clonic seizures. True/False

b. Pyrexia. True/False

c. Labile blood pressure. True/False

d. Flushing. True/False

e. Urinary incontinence. True/False

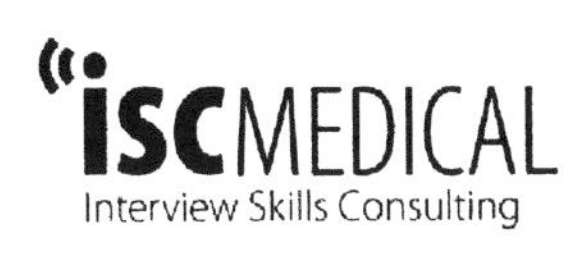

333 The following are short or medium-acting benzodiazepines. **PSYCH**

a. Temazepam. True/False

b. Lorazepam. True/False

c. Chlordiazepoxide. True/False

d. Diazepam. True/False

e. Oxazepam. True/False

334 The following patients would not tend to do well in group therapy. **PSYCH**

a. Those with severe depression. True/False

b. Schizoid personality types. True/False

c. A mother grieving the death of her infant from sudden infant death syndrome. True/False

d. Narcissistic personality types. True/False

e. Bipolar patient in a manic episode. True/False

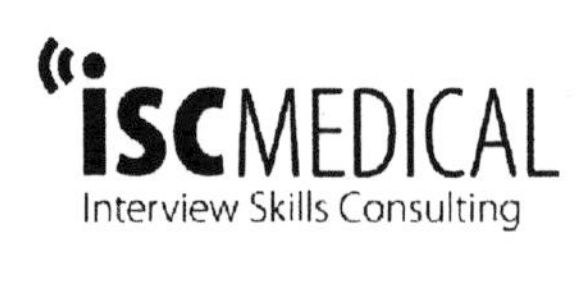

335	The following is true regarding obsessive compulsive disorder (OCD).	PSYCH

a. An obsession can be a word, thought or image. True/False

b. The person who experiences the obsession knows that the obsession is unreal or that it makes no sense. True/False

c. Mild cases is often treated with SSRIs alone. True/False

d. Ritualistic behaviour is noted in OCD. True/False

e. Compulsions often involve somatisation behaviour. True/False

336	The following is true regarding psychotherapy.	PSYCH

a. Cognitive therapy has been found to be of use for alcohol abuse. True/False

b. Counselling involves listening and reflecting on a patients problems and generating a strategy with advice for what to do next. True/False

c. Psycho-analytical therapy involves talking through and making links from experiences from earlier life events. True/False

d. Supportive psychotherapy is therapy that is used in addition to or supports other techniques e.g. cognitive or behavioural therapies. True/False

e. Cognitive behavioural therapy reduces the relapse rate in treated depression. True/False

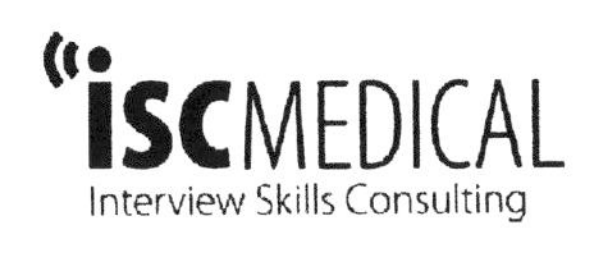

337	Seasonal affective disorder.	PSYCH

a. Hyperphagia is far more common than in other depressive episodes. True/False

b. Light therapy correlates with suppressed plasma melatonin. True/False

c. Is related to melatonin production from the hypothalamus. True/False

d. Light from the ultra-violet end of the visual spectrum has been shown to be most effective in treatment. True/False

e. Is more common in women than men. True/False

338	The following are accepted criteria in the diagnosis of anorexia nervosa.	PSYCH

a. Amenorrhoea. True/False

b. Lack of self esteem. True/False

c. Excessive exercise. True/False

d. Disturbance of body image. True/False

e. Fear of becoming obese. True/False

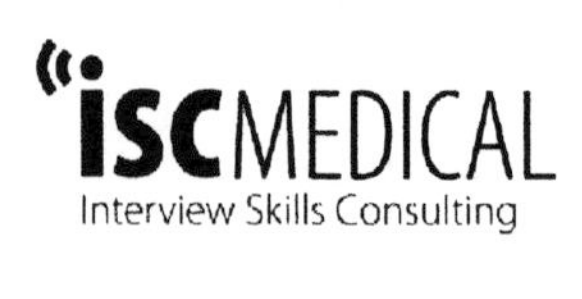

339 The following are recognised physical sequelae of anorexia nervosa. **PSYCH**

a. Alopecia. True/False

b. Steatorrhoea. True/False

c. Hypotension. True/False

d. Cardiac arrest from dysrhythmia. True/False

e. Growth of lanugo hairs. True/False

340 Regarding anorexia nervosa. **PSYCH**

a. Bingeing on food makes the diagnosis very unlikely. True/False

b. One should be aware of sexual abuse in the family which is highly associated with anorexia nervosa. True/False

c. Enteral or parenteral feeding is rarely indicated. True/False

d. Almost all patients will have normalised their weight after 4 or 5 years of professional help. True/False

e. Anorexia has the highest death rate of any psychiatric disorder. True/False

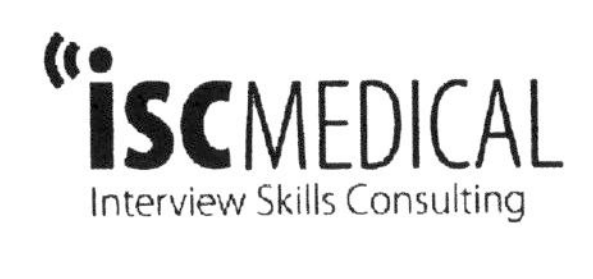

341 The following are recognised criteria in the diagnosis of bulimia nervosa. **PSYCH**

a. Binge eating. True/False

b. Eating more than 3 meals per day. True/False

c. Disturbance of self perceived body weight. True/False

d. Excessive use of purgatives. True/False

e. Preoccupation with body weight. True/False

342 The following is true regarding new or 'atypical' antipsychotics. **PSYCH**

a. They are becoming first line agents in children. True/False

b. They risk agranulocytosis. True/False

c. Cigarette smoking increases their drug levels. True/False

d. They are useful in the treatment of the negative symptoms of schizophrenia. True/False

e. They have no risk in the development of neuroleptic malignant syndrome. True/False

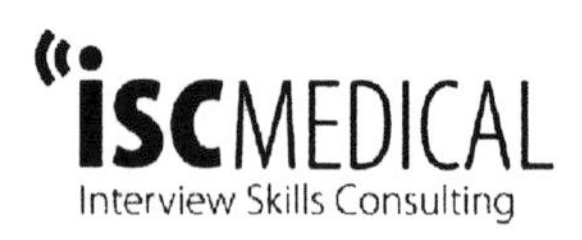

343	The following are contraindications to the use of electroconvulsive therapy.	PSYCH

a. Previous haemorrhagic or ischaemic stroke. True/False

b. Negative symptoms in schizophrenia. True/False

c. Use of atypical antipsychotics. True/False

d. Febrile convulsions as a child. True/False

e. Raised intracranial pressure. True/False

344	The following are characteristic of post traumatic stress disorder.	PSYCH

a. Features typically within in one year of a stressful event. True/False

b. Compulsive behaviours. True/False

c. Reliving of previous events. True/False

d. Tearfulness. True/False

e. Increased startle response. True/False

345 Tricyclic antidepressants. **PSYCH**

a. Tricyclics are the best option if suicide risk is high. True/False

b. Tricyclics are contraindicated in the elderly. True/False

c. Overall tricyclics are less effective than SSRIs. True/False

d. Tricyclics are intolerable in children and so are best avoided. True/False

e. Tricyclics are of value during pregnancy and breast feeding. True/False

346 The following are associated with a good prognosis in schizophrenia. **PSYCH**

a. Absence of negative symptoms. True/False

b. Presence of affective symptoms. True/False

c. Abnormalities on CT. True/False

d. Gradual onset of symptoms. True/False

e. Absence of precipitating stressors. True/False

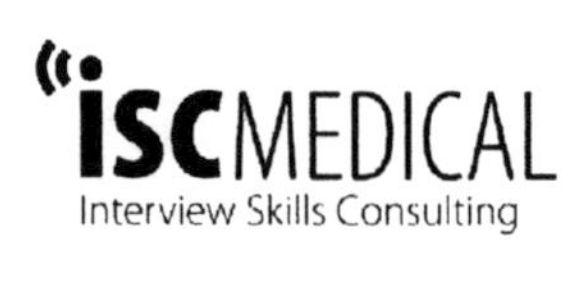

347 The following is true regarding antidepressants. **PSYCH**

a. Antidepressant side effects generally take a week to present. True/False

b. Antidepressants are often contraindicated in multiple sclerosis. True/False

c. Antidepressants can increase risk of glaucoma. True/False

d. An improvement tends to begin around 3 weeks after starting antidepressant treatment. True/False

e. SSRIs can often be stopped completely within two weeks after restoration of mood. True/False

348 The following are recognised side effects of SSRIs. **PSYCH**

a. Hyperpyrexia syndrome. True/False

b. Disorders of ejaculation. True/False

c. Malignant hypertension. True/False

d. Tardive dyskinesia. True/False

e. Akathisia. True/False

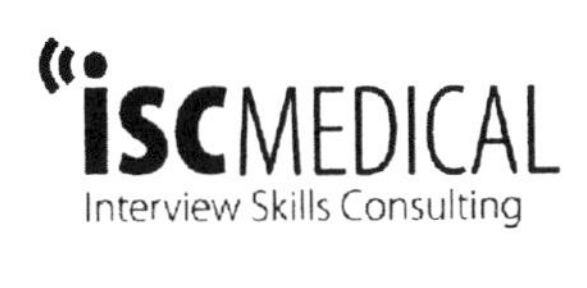

349 The following are indications for the use of electroconvulsive therapy. **PSYCH**

a. Obsessive compulsive disorder. True/False

b. Schizoaffective disorder. True/False

c. Mania. True/False

d. Catatonic schizophrenia. True/False

e. Anorexia nervosa. True/False

350 Electroconvulsive therapy (ECT). **PSYCH**

a. Treatment usually consists of 8 to 12 sessions. True/False

b. Patients are often reassured by witnessing the procedure on other patients before undertaking it themselves. True/False

c. Benzodiazepines are contraindicated, before, during and after the procedure since they increase the seizure threshold and render it ineffective. True/False

d. Efficacy is related to the length of seizure produced. True/False

e. Glaucoma is a relative contraindication. True/False

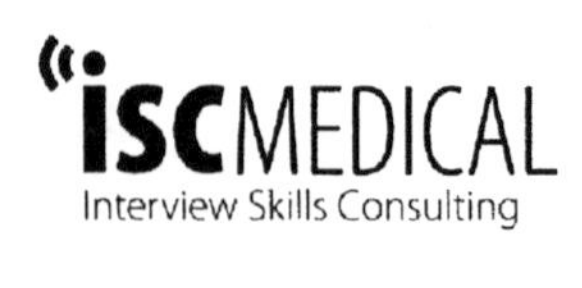

351 The follow conditions are recognised causes of Wernicke-Korsakoff syndrome. **PSYCH**

a. Pernicious anaemia. True/False

b. Gastric carcinoma. True/False

c. Cocaine abuse. True/False

d. Abuse of emetics. True/False

e. Pregnancy. True/False

352 The following conditions are correctly matched with their definitions. **PSYCH**

a. Dysmorphophobia : Fear of becoming disfigured. True/False

b. Hypochondriasis : A subtype of somatoform disorder in which the patient is preoccupied with the concern that they have a medical illness. True/False

c. Neurasthenia : An old term for what is now called chronic fatigue syndrome. True/False

d. Somatisation : A patient complains of loss of function (e.g. of a limb) where there is no physical problem identifiable. True/False

e. Dissociative disorder : A patient complains of symptoms for which there is no medical explanation e.g. chronic pain. True/False

353 The following types of personality disorder are correctly matched with their descriptions. **PSYCH**

a. Borderline : Close to anxiety disorder, with continued apprehension and avoidance of others for fear of rejection. True/False
b. Narcissistic : Stubborn and humourless, like to perform in front of an audience. True/False
c. Anankastic : Multiple turbulent relationships, unstable mood and impulsivity. True/False
d. Histrionic : Theatrical expressions of emotion, vain and attention seeking. True/False
e. Schizoid : Suspicious and distrusting of others, self important and stubborn. True/False

354 The following is true regarding the Mental Health Act 1983. **PSYCH**

a. Both doctors who sign the 'Section 2' must be 'approved' under the mental health act. True/False

b. Section 2 is applicable to a patient with severe depression who needs admission for heparin for a large DVT, but who is refusing because they know it could kill them if left untreated. True/False

c. Section 5(2) applies to a patient in hospital who must be detained e.g. a psychotic self harmer who arrives in A&E. True/False

d. In a section 5(4) a nurse may hold a patient for up to 12 hours whilst other medical and psychiatric staff are assembled to convert to a section 5, e.g. a patient on a general surgical ward who wants to leave post-operatively. True/False

e. Section 4 lasts for up to 72 hours and is for emergency treatment. A GP and a close relative are all that are needed for this. True/False

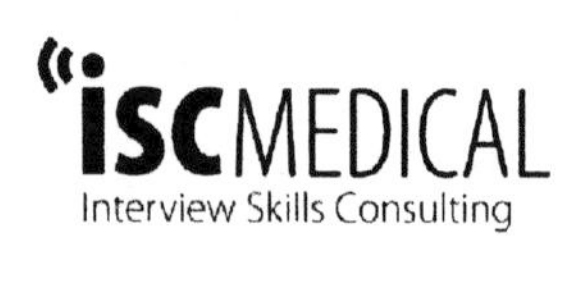

355 The following is true of epilepsy and pregnancy. **PSYCH**

a. Epilepsy in the pregnant woman is associated with an increase risk of premature delivery. True/False

b. Foetal facial abnormalities are increased if the mother has epilepsy in pregnancy even without taking anticonvulsants. True/False

c. A significant number of newborns born to epileptic mother will experience symptoms due to anticonvulsant withdrawal after birth. True/False

d. Folic acid supplements should be given to babies after delivery. True/False

e. Autism risk is increased in those who had been exposed to certain types of anticonvulsants during pregnancy. True/False

356 The following features are suggestive of autism in a child. **PSYCH**

a. Has few friends of his/her own age despite good interaction with older siblings and cousins. True/False

b. Is reluctant to be comforted when physically hurt. True/False

c. A girl preferring to play with trucks and bricks than dollies. True/False

d. Obsessive collection of unusual objects e.g. all the bus tickets he/she has ever used. True/False

e. Muddling of pronouns when speaking. True/False

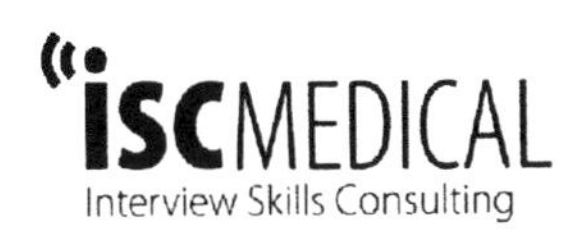

357 The following features may be seen in childhood depression. **PSYCH**

a. Antisocial behaviour. True/False

b. Excessive sleepiness. True/False

c. Somnambulance. True/False

d. Truancy. True/False

e. Complaints of boredom. True/False

358 The following are correct definitions of techniques used in psychotherapy. **PSYCH**

a. Avoidance is a technique in behavioural therapy which allows a patient to distance themselves from situations of potential anxiety. True/False

b. Systematic desensitisation is a technique in sex therapy where one gradually increases a stimulus to become more and more used to it. True/False

c. Sensate focus is a technique used in sex therapy to do with focusing on non-genital areas of stimulation. True/False

d. Flooding is a technique used in psychoanalytic therapy where one clears ones minds or floods ones thoughts of emotion. True/False

e. Graded exposure is a cognitive technique where one slowly recounts a scenario or vignette and bit by bit identifies sources of anxiety. True/False

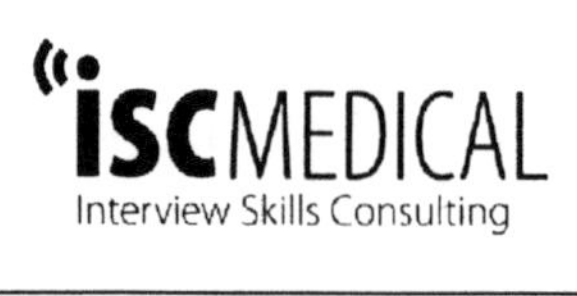

359	The following is true regarding Alzheimer's dementia.	PSYCH

a. Risk is increased in those with cystic fibrosis. True/False

b. People using NSAIDs have a reduced risk of developing Alzheimer's dementia. True/False

c. Ginkgo biloba is beneficial in reducing the risk of developing Alzheimer's dementia. True/False

d. Average time from diagnosis to death is around 4 years. True/False

e. It is associated with loss of noradrenergic activity in the temporal lobes. True/False

360	The following are features of high risk associated with a suicide attempt.	PSYCH

a. Presence of a suicide note. True/False

b. Suicide attempted in a secluded place. True/False

c. Alcohol consumption at time of the event. True/False

d. The person preparing their finances beforehand. True/False

e. Use of a firearm. True/False

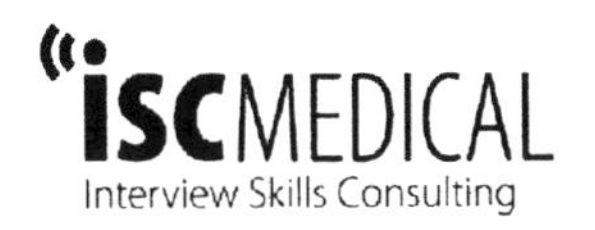

MCQs for GPVTS

ANSWERS

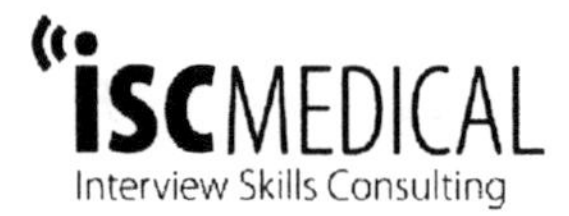

1 **TTTTF**
Most strawberry naevi can be left and they will regress spontaneously.

2 **TFFFT**
Stems b and c are unproven.

3 **TFTTF**

4 **TFFTF**
Erysipelas is strep whilst impetigo is staph. Stem c describes impetigo which occurs mainly on the face.

5 **FFFFF**
A 'black-head' is due to the oxydation of trapped sebum in contact with air. Initial treatments include drying the skin and so emollients may make matters worse.

6 **FTFTF**
Oral and topical antibiotics should be the same type to avoid the development of resistant bacteria. Antibiotic treatment may be considered but a course of between 6 weeks' and 6 months' duration is usually required to initiate and sustain improvement.

7 **TFTTF**
Comedones are absent.

8 **FTTFF**
Wickham's striae are not restricted to mucosal lesions.

9 **TTFTF**
In pemphigoid, it is linear IgG that is seen. For stem e the opposite is true.

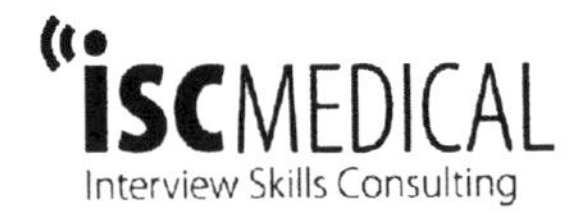

10 **TTFFT**

ECM is associated with Lyme disease and Livedo reticularis with antiphospholipid syndrome.

11 **TTTTF**

Symptoms do not appear until a type IV immune response has developed to proteins excreted by the mites. The whole household must be treated simultaneously. Animal scabies does exist but it is rarely transmitted to humans and is short-lived if it does. Pets are only treated when fleas are diagnosed.

12 **FFTFT**

Telangectasia is a complication of topical steroids but mild steroids aren't contraindicated on the face. TH2 cells and IgE are implicated in this type I hypersensitivity. Nickel is part of a type IV or 'Allergic contact' dermatitis. S.Aureus is potentially responsible for superantigens which are involved with the pathogenesis of atopic dermatitis.

13 **TTTTF**

HHV8 is implicated in Kaposi's sarcoma.

14 **TTTTT**

15 **TTFFF**

16 **TTTFT**

Infliximab not Rituximab is the monoclonal antibody of use. UVA with psoralen (PUVA) is also used (e.g. for large plaques).

17 **FTTFT**

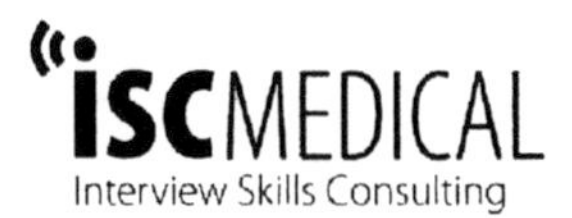

18 **FTTTT**

Lichenification is a reaction to excessive scratching as a sign of an underlying disease rather than a disease that occurs at a site of injury. It is controversial as to whether Molluscum do 'Köbnerise' or whether it is really auto-inoculation of the pox virus from site to site.

19 **TTFTT**

Acanthosis nigricans is associated with pancreatic carcinoma. Tylosis hyperkeratosis of the soles and palms and is associated with oesophageal carcinoma.

20 **FTTFF**

All of these have been linked to erythema multiforme but only amoxicillin and mycoplasma are relatively common causative factors.

21 **TTTTF**

Lesions tend to have raised or 'shouldered' edges and central cratering.

22 **FTTTT**

23 **FTTFF**

The factor is how much longer one can stay in the sun before burning. Skin type 1 individuals tend to take care in the sun because they burn so easily. Skin types 1 and 2 are the fairest and most prone to melanoma.

24 **FTTTT**

25 **TTTTF**

26 **FTTTF**

Dithranol should be applied for 20 minutes or so, then washed off and it is best to avoid the eyes.

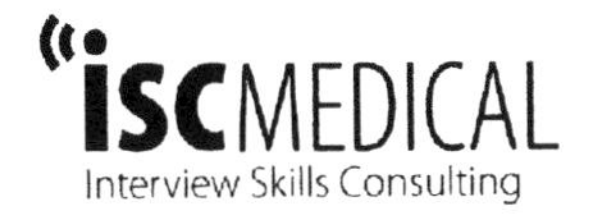

27 **TFTFF**

28 **TTTFT**

29 **TFFFT**

RAST looks for IgE which is pivotal in type 1 hypersensitivity. Use of steroid sprays in unlimited. It is decongestants that lead to a rebound phenomenon.

30 **FTFTT**

The top third of the nose is bony and can be fractured. A skull X-ray is unhelpful in many cases since soft tissue oedema may obscure the bony structures.

31 **FTTTF**

Crack cocaine is smoked not snorted.

32 **TTTTT**

33 **TFTTT**

Discharge is often watery from the nostril but purulent if postnasal.

34 **FFTFT**

The head should be kept forward to prevent posterior drip. The cartilage not the bony bridge must be pinched. Packing is often indicated when the bleeding site is not seen.

35 **TFTTT**

Most cases of acute sinusitis do not require antibiotics. Decongestants and steaming may be all that is required.

36 **TFFFT**

Tonsillitis is usually due to a group A streptococcus. Haemorrhage in the first 24 hours post operatively requires operative intervention, whereas after 5 days it is usually due to infection and surgery is rarely required.

37 **FTFTF**

More than 5 attacks per year for more than 5 days over a 2 year period is one accepted guideline.

38 **TTTFF**

39 **TTFTT**

Attacks usually occur after 5 to 10 seconds following sudden head movement. The vertigo persist for about 30 to 60 seconds. Laser ablation is really a last resort therapy.

40 **FTFTT**

41 **TTTFT**

42 **TTTTT**

43 **TFFTT**

RLN palsy can be caused by aortic aneurysm but not coarctation itself, although it is a complication of surgical repair.

44 **TTFFF**

This can be congenital or acquired. It can follow ear drum perforation or just with otherwise uncomplicated otitis media. Cholesterol is not involved at all.

45 **TFTTT**

Chondrodermatitis nodularis is a painful condition that can be treated with excision. Wax production is confined to the outer third of the canal.

46 **TTTFF**

Sentence structure and word order are of concern at 5 years of age.

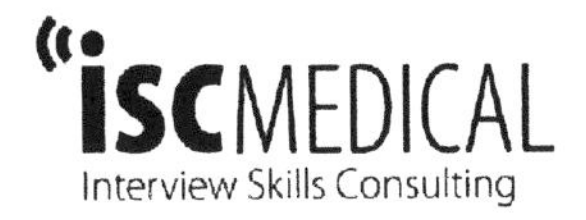

47 **TTTFT**
A voice prosthesis is required after laryngeal treatment.

48 **FTTFF**
Speech audiometry is also subjective, depending on the patient's verbal responses. Tympanometry assesses the function of the tympanic membrane and the pressure of the middle ear, but cannot assess the integrity of the auditory nerve.

49 **TFTTT**

50 **TFFTT**
The effect of grommets is more sophisticated than simple fluid drainage. Allowing air conduction of sound is implicated.

51 **TFTTF**
Mycoplasma species and viruses are implicated.

52 **TFFTF**

53 **FTTFT**
The halo sign suggests CSF in the fluid (it occurs when the fluid containing both blood and CSF is placed on filter paper. The blood remains as a central spot and CSF diffuses outwards). Blood in discharge can be due to many causes including trauma to the external ear and ear canal.

54 **TTTTT**

55 **TTTTT**
Osteosclerosis appears to be an autosomal dominant condition with variable penetrance. It may be worsened by pregnancy or the Pill.

56 **TFTFT**

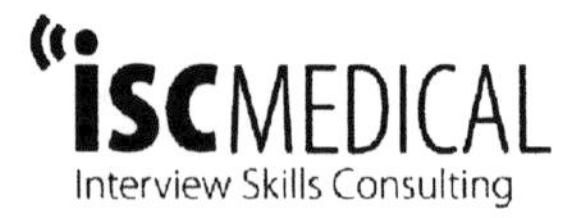

57 **FTTFT**

Loop diuretics are implicated.

58 **TFTFF**

59 **TFTFT**

Otitis externa tends to be a separate condition from furunculosis. Pseudomonal agents are implicated in otitis externa and so gentamicin and steroid drops are often used. Furunculosis is generally treated conservatively.

60 **TTTFT**

61 **FFTTT**

These glands are a 'normal' finding and occasionally block with or without infection. If surgery is indicated (severe cases), they are drained and marsupialised.

62 **TTTTT**

63 **FTTTT**

Topical oestrogens are a treatment for post-menopausal atrophic vaginitis, the symptoms of which may include localised irritation.

64 **TFTTF**

20% of complete moles subsequently progress to invasive disease, and monitoring of b-HCG is vital. Pregnancy should be avoided so that recurrence can be detected with elevated b-HCG. Fortunately, there is an excellent response to chemotherapy.

65 **TFTTF**

Laparoscopy is preferred due to the faster recovery time. Salpingotomy runs the risk of a retained trophoblast and subsequent ectopic pregnancies so it is reserved for those with only one functioning tube.

66 **FTFFT**

67 **FFTTT**

Ectopic pregnancies account for 0.25%-1% of pregnancies; the rate is higher in some countries were sexually transmitted infections are more prevalent. A pregnancy test and an ultrasound should be performed if these is any suspicion of a possible ectopic pregnancy.

68 **FFTFF**

69 **FTFFT**

Missed abortion is when the foetus dies but is retained. Threatened abortion is early pregnancy bleeding, when the os is closed and 3/4 will settle. Inevitable abortion is early pregnancy bleeding with an open cervical os.

70 **TFTTT**

Only severe PID needs inpatient management a lot is dealt with in primary care and via GUM clinics.

71 **FFTFT**

The pill, cervical cap and pregnancy are protective.

72 **FTTFF**

Many are asymptomatic or are treated with medication alone. Deposits may rarely go beyond the peritoneum (lung). It affects up to 12% of women.

73 **FFFTT**

The transformation zone is the border or the columnar endocervix with the squamous ectocervix. Cervical polyps are benign but are excised if symptoms (bleeding or discharge) are present. Nabothian cysts are harmless and need not be reviewed.

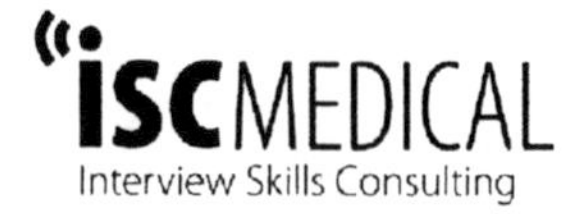

74 **TTTFF**

Semen should not be kept below 12 degrees celsius. Hysterosalpingogram is invasive and many other tests including hormone profile precede it.

75 **TTFFT**

76 **FFTFF**

Artificial insemination by donor is of use when partner sperm count is low otherwise laboratory techniques are required. Success rates are variable between clinics, from 10%-50% per cycle, and also vary with maternal age. The national average is around 20% success per cycle.

77 **FTTFF**

Spermicides must be used with other devices if they are to have a significant reduction in pregnancy. Timing of coitus is effective at reducing pregnancy but not very reliable. Ejaculation outside the vagina is not easily reproducible and the cervix may still be exposed to pre-ejaculate material which contain viable spermatozoa. The teat on the condom MUST be squeezed to allow later expansion with filling to avoid splitting.

78 **FTFTF**

On average most IUCD are changed 3 to 5 yearly.

79 **FFTFT**

EC is 95% effective in 24hours, 85% up to 48 hours and 58% up to 72 hour. A doctor can still prescribe it beyond 72 hours but the effectiveness is much reduced.

80 **TTFFT**

A cardiac risk factor is a relative contraindication, two or more is absolute. Active hepatic disease is an absolute contraindication.

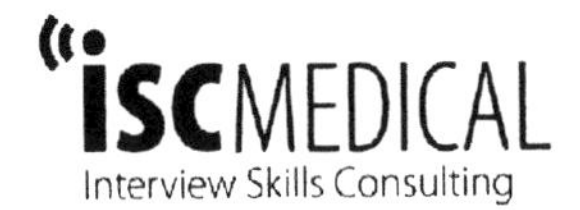

81 **TFFFT**

Antibiotics such as rifampicin may reduce the effectiveness of the COCP by enzyme reduction, but for other antibiotics the effect is much smaller and appears to be due to change in gut flora reducing gut recycling of ethinyestradiol. Barrier contraception should be advised for 7 days (sometimes longer) after the liver enzyme inducing drug is stopped. PoP has no problems with stroke risk like COCP. COCP is absolutely contraindicated in migraine with aura. If no aura, it can be given as long as there are no other stroke risk factors. Penicillins are not noted as liver enzyme inducers (Tetracyclines are).

82 **TFFFT**

Main mode of action is by making cervical mucus hostile to sperm. It must be taken strictly to time each day to maintain effective drug levels and therefore it is not reliable in those with chaotic lives. The exception to stem b is Cerazette ® which is the only PoP that suppresses ovulation.

83 **FTTFF**

Depot is given 3 monthly. Implants are changed usually every 3 years and their contraceptive cover immediately stops once removed.

84 **TFTFT**

Diaphragms come in a variety of sizes and must be individually chosen for each patient. The contraceptive effect of the progestogens implant is immediately reversed upon the removal of the implant. However, some women may experience a delay in return to fertility for up to one year following their last depot injection.

85 **TTFFF**

Smears show dyskaryosis, a reflection of CIN. CIN is a histological diagnosis made after biopsy. Time between smears increases to five years from three at 50 but does not stop until 65. CIN can progress but also revert to earlier stages.

86 **TTFFT**

BV causes problems later in pregnancy as does cervical incompetence.

87 **FTFTT**

Urethrocele leads to stress incontinence. Ring pessaries are mainly a temporary measure prior to surgical intervention at a later date. They may be permanent in those unsuitable for pelvic surgery.

88 **TTTTT**

89 **TTTFT**

Early onset of coitus is associated.

90 **FFTFF**

Pre TOP ultrasound is performed in many but not all centres unfortunately. Medical abortion is used until week 9. Up to 5% of medically treated TOPs will go on to require surgical evacuation.

91 **FTTTT**

Rarely, TOPs are performed after 24 weeks if there is risk of grave injury to mother or risk of serious disability in the newborn.

92 **FFFTT**

The patches only contain the oestrogen. Progesterone must be given orally to those with a uterus. Family history would have to be probed further and risks and benefits of HRT weighed up before it is discounted. Varicose veins are linked to deep venous incompetence and thrombo-embolism. After five years of use, the risks of breast cancers begin to rise.

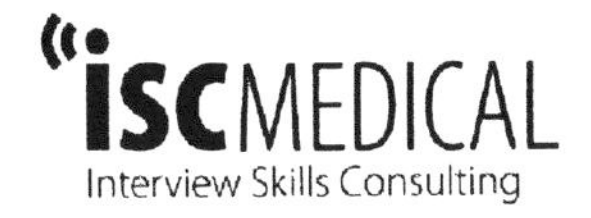

93 **TFTTT**

Ovarian tumours tend to present late. They can cause mass effects directly or due to lymphadenopathy which can obstruct the ureters.

94 **TFFTF**

HRT can increase risk of any oestrogen dependent tumour. Progesterone should be given when an endometrium is present. Protects against osteoporosis but not cardiovascular disease (current evidence).

95 **TFTTT**

96 **FTFFT**

Overt carcinoma is most often picked up due to presenting symptoms. Sexual intercourse is recommended post radiotherapy to prevent stricturing and stenosis. Smears after radiotherapy are uninterpretable and of no value.

97 **FFFTT**

DUB is most often the cause in young women. Mefanamic acid reduces the pain of dysmenorrhoea whilst tranexamic acid reduces blood loss. COCP should not be considered in women over 35 years or smokers.

98 **TFFFT**

HRT should be used with caution in women with lupus or hypertension but many such women use it with no problem. Antiphospholipid syndrome is a contraindication because of the high risk of thromboembolus.

99 **TTTTF**

Psychotherapy is beneficial in cases related to anorexia where it may allow the body mass index to rise above a critical point for ovulation to occur.

100 **FTTFT**
Referral should always be made if bleeding occurs more than 12 months after the final period.

101 **FFFFT**
A small percentage of cervical cancer is caused by adenocarcinoma (not squamous cell) and so is not associated with HPV.

102 **FFTTF**

103 **FFTFT**

104 **TTTTT**

105 **FFFTF**
Prevalence is 20%.

106 **TTFFT**
Lowering saturated fats has been shown to decrease the oestrogen interaction with its receptors.

107 **FTTTT**
Mucinous cystadenomas lead to pseudomyxoma peritonei. Fibromas commonly lead to Meig's syndrome.

108 **TTTFF**
Raloxifene has no effect on hot flushes.

109 **FTTTF**

110 **TTFTT**
Although BV is not a sexually transmitted infection, the pH of the vagina may be elevated by the presence of sperm and this may disrupt the balance of flora normally maintained by Lactobacilli and allow Gardnerella to flourish.

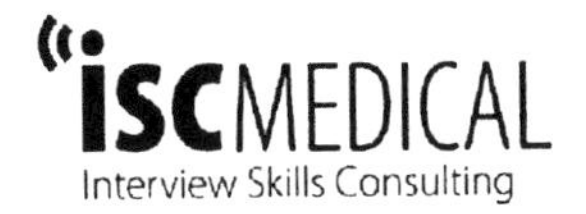

111 **TFTFF**

112 **TTTTT**

113 **TFTTT**

114 **FFFTT**

Oral contraceptives have poor response rates. Many women have fibroids, with no need for treatment. Red degeneration is treated with analgesia and rest. Torsion is a surgical emergency.

115 **TFFTT**

If fibroids are large enough to cause a significant pelvic obstruction to venous return from the lower limbs, risk of deep vein thrombosis can be increased.

116 **TFTTT**

117 **TTFFF**

118 **FFTTF**

119 **TFFFF**

The membranes are often ruptured artificially. Induction is not contraindicated for breech delivery but is rarely used as the majority are delivered by elective caesarian section. Augmentation should not be used.

120 **FFTTT**

121 **TTTFF**

It is defined as fluid >2 litres in volume. Indomethacin, not prostaglandins, are useful in this condition.

122 **FTTFT**

123 **TTFFF**

124 **FTTTF**

H2 blockers are given to reduce the risks of aspiration if a seizure should occur. Steroids are given if preterm delivery appears inevitable.

125 **FTFTT**

Kick charts register concern if kicks are fewer than 10 per day. Foetal bradycardia is rarely associated with hypoxia.

126 **FFTFT**

Rubella screening identifies those women who would benefit from vaccination after delivery. The vaccine is a live vaccine and should not be given within 3 months of subsequent pregnancy. Only half of women are symptomatic.

127 **FTTFT**

Stroke is the most common cause of death.

128 **TTTTT**

129 **FTFTT**

Nitrazine sticks can suggest but not diagnose presence of liquor, since there are many false positives (blood, alkaline urine, semen or vaginal infection). Delaying delivery allows time for the foetus to mature (with steroids) however the disadvantage is the increasing risk of infection as time passes.

130 **FTFTT**

Heparin can be given is an epidural is sited, but it is restricted to specific timing away from lumbar puncture and catheter removal. Urinary retention not incontinence is a complication. Intravenous fluid infusion is used to counteract the postural hypotension which is a complication of epidural anaesthesia.

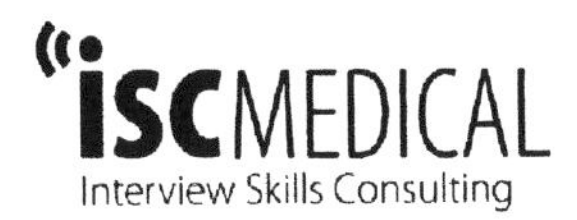

131 **TTFTF**
Steroids are of value if given more than 24 hours before delivery.

132 **FTFFF**
This equates to hypoxia and acidosis. Foetal pH is tested by foetal blood sampling.

133 **FFTTT**
It is delivery beyond 42 weeks.

134 **FTTFT**

135 **TFTTT**

136 **FTTFT**

137 **FFFTT**
These drugs abate uterine contractions to avert or delay labour.

138 **TTFTT**

139 **FFFFF**

140 **TFTTF**

141 **FTFTF**
The most common type of breech is the 'extended' type with buttocks presenting and the knees extended. ECV is performed at around 34 - 36 weeks. Forceps are sometimes but certainly not always used.

142 **FFFTF**
Whilst stems a, c and e may indicate caesarean section, only uterine fibroids from the list may indicate a 'classical' vertical incision section from the much more common lower segment incision.

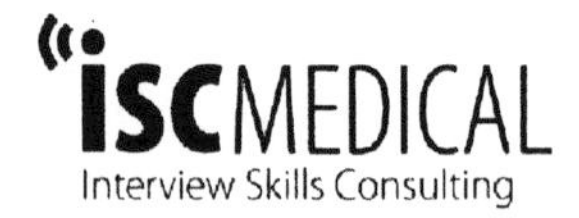

143 FFFTT

Theophylines are used to reduce bronchospasm, but in established cases and not as prophylaxis. Sodium citrate is taken enterally. H2 antagonists are most commonly used preoperatively.

144 FTTTF

145 TFTTT

Pre-eclampsia can lead to hepatic congestion causing pain.

146 FFFFT

Stillbirth includes death in utero and refers to any baby born dead after 24 weeks gestation. Induction tends not to include amniotomy due to theoretical infection risk. Risk of DIC is rare before 3 weeks post foetal death. Post mortem may be refused by the parents.

147 FTTFT

Those factors which decrease uterine contractions also lead to decreased contractions of dilated vessels which would otherwise continue to bleed post partum.

148 TTTFT

149 TTFFF

Amniocentesis leads to miscarriage is around 1% of cases.

150 TTFFT

Squamous cells seen in lung tissue in the mother is a post mortem finding. Hypotension is corrected by fluid resuscitation to a normal blood pressure after which further fluids are carefully given.

151 FTFTT

Risk of uterine rupture is increased in second and subsequent pregnancies especially with the use of oxytocin.

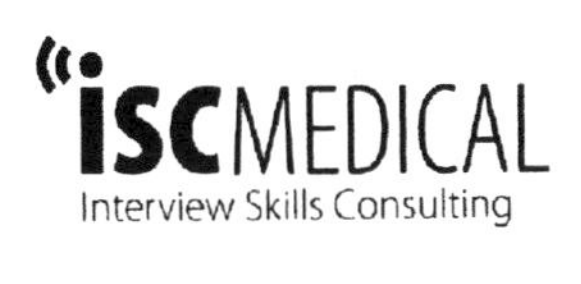

152 **TTFTT**
Antiphospholipid syndrome gives predominantly first trimester loss.

153 **FTFTT**

154 **TFTFF**

155 **FTTTF**

156 **TFFTT**

157 **TTFTF**
Colostrum persists for 3 days post partum. The uterus takes about 10 days to shrink down into the pelvis.

158 **FTTTT**

159 **TTTTF**

160 **TFTTT**

161 **TTFTT**
Oral hypoglycaemics are contraindicated if the mother intends to breast feed. Since not all women do breast feed, this cannot be a generalised rule.

162 **FTFTT**
Radioactive iodine is contraindicated during pregnancy and lactation.

163 **FTTFT**

164 **TTFFF**
Ankle oedema, calf pain and pruritus are very common in pregnancy and should not cause alarm in the majority of patients.

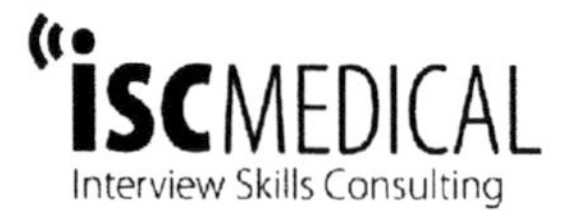

165 **FFFFT**
A chignon is a phenomenon seen following ventouse delivery. The cervix must be fully dilated as a prerequisite for use.

166 **TTFFT**

167 **FFFTF**
Gravida refers to the number of pregnancies including any current ones. With 'Para a+b', a= number of pregnancies beyond 24 weeks whether live or stillborn; b=number of pregnancies terminated or miscarried prior to 24 weeks.

168 **TTTFF**

169 **TTTFT**

170 **TTFFF**
Normal rate is around 3 every 10 minutes.

171 **TFTTF**

172 **FFFTT**
SFH is measured in cm. Age in weeks roughly equals SFH +/- a few cms with progression of the pregnancy.

173 **FTTTT**

174 **FTFFF**

175 **FFTTT**
Cord lengthening is a sign of impending placental delivery in the third stage.

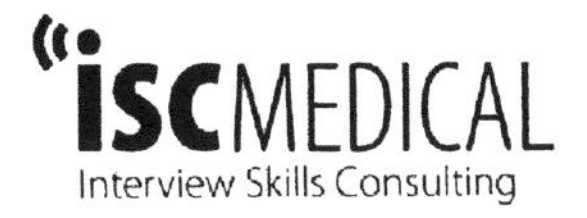

176 **TFTFF**
Vaginal exam for cervical dilatation is due every 4 hours. Foetal heart rate is measured every 15 minutes. Maternal vital signs are measure half hourly.

177 **TFFFT**
A pregnancy test generally remains positive until around the 20th week of pregnancy.

178 **TTFFT**
Total cortisol rises but free levels remain constant. Prolactin rises throughout pregnancy.

179 **FTFFF**
About 3% of early identified low lying placentas result in a placenta previa at term.

180 **FFTTF**
AR pupils are also found in diabetes. The Marcus Gunn pupil will dilate when a light is shone at it. The Holmes-Aide pupil does react to stimuli, it is just slow or "sluggish".

181 **FTTTF**

182 **FTTTT**

183 **FTFFF**
Ulcerative keratitis involves ulceration, keratitis alone is just inflammation of the cornea. Herpes simplex causes dendritic ulcers. Many types of infective agents as well as non infective conditions cause keratitis and ulceration hence a low threshold for further management involving an ophthalmologist should be encouraged.

184 **FFTTT**

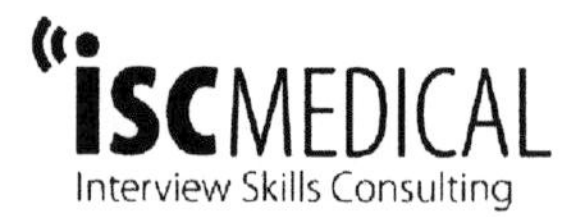

185 **TTTFT**

A pseudo squint is an illusion of discordant eye gaze due to wide epicanthic folds. Squints should be promptly referred to an ophthalmologist since a delay may lead to loss of vision in the affected eye.

186 **FFTTF**

The red reflex is often lost or attenuated, not potentiated. This is a tumour that occurs in young children and often from birth. Hence it may well be picked up on childhood screening and certainly before the child is able to complain of visual disturbance.

187 **FFTTF**

Around 20% of shingles is ophthalmic.

188 **FTTFF**

189 **TTFFT**

Keratoconjunctivitis sicca is the formal name for dry eyes. This is most commonly attributed to old age. Schirmer's test is used. Schober's test is used to evaluate restriction of axial movement in ankylosing spondylitis.

190 **TTFTF**

An ectropion is an eversion of an eye lid. A pinguela is on the conjunctiva not the cornea. If it encroaches the cornea, it is termed a pterygium.

191 **FTFTT**

Scleritis tends to be deeper and more often related to connective tissue disorders. It is also scleritis (not episcleritis) which leads to perforation of the globe.

192 **TTTTF**

Latanoprost increases outflow of aqueous.

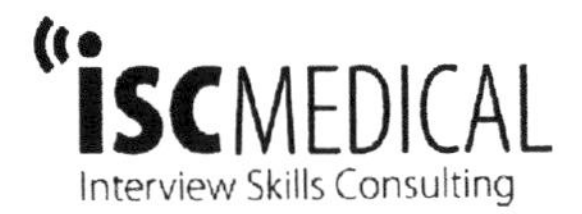

193 **TTFTT**

Keratomalacia is related to vitamin A deficiency and so also night blindness. The cornea is dry and can perforate. Vitamin A supplementation is contraindicated in pregnancy. Chlamydia trachomatic serovars A-C cause trachoma and D-K cause genital tract infections.

194 **TFTFT**

Angioid streaks are breaks in Buchs membrane associated with connective tissue diseases.

195 **FFTTT**

Mild background retinopathy can be monitored regularly in a diabetic clinic. Maculopathy warrants urgent referral. Rubeosis can lead to glaucoma.

196 **FFTTF**

Type 1 diabetics usually have 5 -10 years from diabetes diagnosis before onset of retinopathy. Maculopathy is more common in type 2 diabetes. Trials have shown that tight glycaemic and blood pressure control are beneficial to all diabetes complications. However, blood pressure control is more often related to macrovascular complications.

197 **FFTTT**

All five are features of preproliferative retinopathy.

198 **TFFTT**

199 **FTFTT**

200 **TTTTF**

201 **FTTTF**

Many patients can resume full activities the day following day-case surgery.

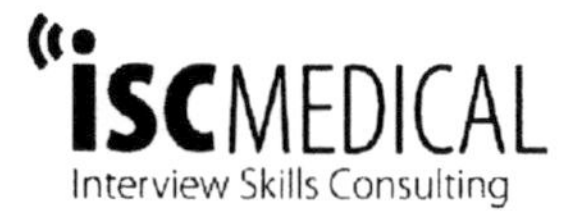

202 **TTFFT**

All of these infections may cause choroidoretinitis but vertically-transmitted HSV and VZV are rare causes.

203 **FTFFT**

The disc cup is widened in glaucoma. Visual loss is a late feature, with acuity being preserved up until irreversible changes have occurred in many patients.

204 **TFTTT**

205 **TFTFT**

206 **FFTTF**

Stem a refers to a temporal lobe lesion. Stem b is likely to refer to retinal pathology such as a branch vein or artery occlusion. Macular sparing occurs when the lesion is confined to the posterior of the occipital lobe.

207 **TTTFT**

The fovea should not be lasered!

208 **FFTFT**

Vitreous haemorrhage may be managed conservatively and, if after many weeks the haemorrhage has not reabsorbed, vitrectomy may be indicated. Temporal arteritis tends to affect the arterial supply to the optic nerve rather than the retina. Optic atrophy as described is more likely to cause a chronic rather than sudden visual loss.

209 **TFTFT**

Subconjunctival haemorrhages are minor self limiting conditions. Hypertension may need to be ruled out.

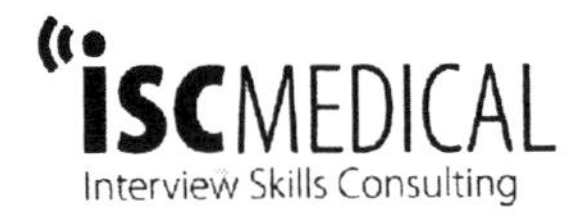

210 **FFTFF**

Chemosis is conjunctival oedema. Keratomalacia is softening of the cornea. Anisocoria is unequal pupil size. Scotoma a defect in part of the visual field.

211 **TTFTF**

212 **TTTFT**

213 **TTTFT**

214 **TFTFT**

Recurrent dislocations involve capsular tears which require surgical repair. Atraumatic dislocations occur in any direction.

215 **FTTTF**

Rheumatoid nodules are a cause of trigger finger. Stem e describes golfer's elbow. Tennis elbow is LATERAL epicondylitis.

216 **TFTTF**

Ankylosis spondylitis more commonly leads to a kyphosis.

217 **FTTFF**

218 **TFFFT**

About half of the patients are obese.

219 **TFTTF**

220 **FFTTF**

T < -1 to -2.5 is osteopenia. T < - 2.5 signifies osteoporosis. T score is not age adjusted, the Z score is.

221 **TFFTF**

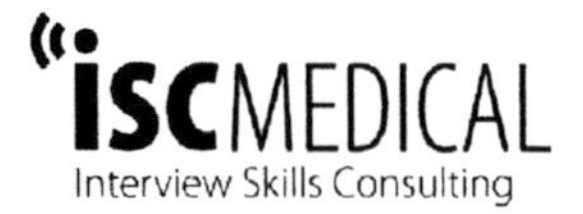

222 FFTFT

Knee effusions and swelling are very commonly associated with osteoarthritis. A Baker's cysts is a herniation of the joint synovium. Joint line tenderness is characteristic of meniscal pathology.

223 TFTFT

224 TTFFF

Barton's fracture is an oblique fracture of the distal radius. Bennett's fracture is a fracture-dislocation of the carpometacarpal joint. Galeazzi fracture is a fracture of the shaft of the radius and dislocation of the distal radio-ulnar joint.

225 TFTTF

Both osteoclastic and osteoblastic activity increase.

226 TFTFT

227 FTFTT

Ultrasound scanning is very useful.

228 TTTFF

Active and passive movement is reduced. Resolution may take several years.

229 TFTFT

230 TFFFF

This is primarily due to a lack of surfactant. Breathing is hard work and laboured. If treatment fails, the baby becomes exhausted, leading to type 2 or ventilatory failure. The symptoms become evident between birth and 4 hours of age. The severity peaks around 48 hours. Although RDS occurs in preterm infants in the significant majority of cases, it is certainly recognised in term infants, especially infants with diabetic mothers.

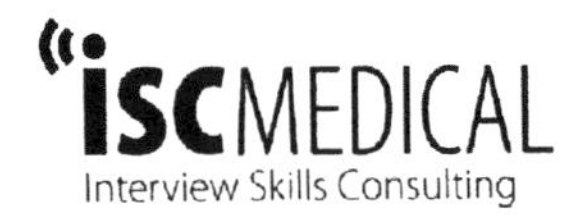

231 **FFTTF**

Elective caesareans don't require paediatric support as a rule. Paediatricians do not routinely go to twin deliveries unless non-cephalic, preterm or section. However they always attend ventouse/forceps deliveries as there is an increased risk of poor condition at birth.

232 **FTFFT**

Ventilation is often all that is needed to reverse acidosis.

233 **TFTTF**

Jaundice under 24 hours is pathological and required investigation for sepsis and haemolysis. From day 2 to 14, jaundice is very common and results from an imbalance between immature liver function and excess red cell destruction. For prolonged jaundice beyond day 14, most cases are still normal "breastfeeding jaundice" but serious causes such a biliary atresia and hypothyroidism must be excluded.

234 **TFTTT**

RoP is caused by fluctuations in oxygen tension in the neonate.

235 **TFFFF**

Single palmar crease may be normal. Per vaginal bleeding is often found as a response to maternal hormones. Most babies with bilateral palmar creases do NOT have Down's syndrome but it should prompt a careful assessment for other features.

236 **TFFTT**

Other features are respiratory effort (cry) and colour.

237 **FFTFF**

A thrill indicates underlying pathology. A VSD murmur is heard loudest at the left sternal edge; sometimes a soft diastolic murmur may also be heard at the apex. A Still's murmur is innocent. A murmur from a PDA is continuous throughout the cardiac cycle.

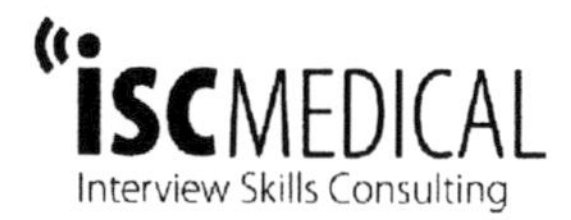

238 **FFFFF**

Any exposure to Rhesus D +ve blood in a Rhesus D –ve mother (including first pregnancy events and sampling procedures) will generate the production of anti-D IgG which can cross the placenta to the foetus. In small amounts this may not cause severe disease in the foetus. Subsequent pregnancies carry an increasing risk of significant amounts of IgG transfer and subsequent harm to the foetus. IgG persists in the neonate after delivery and so this risk is not over after this point.

239 **TFFTF**

Reflex anoxic seizures do not require anticonvulsants as they are initiated by a brief pause in cardiac contractions from vagal overactivity. Infantile spasms involve repetitive jerks that are sometimes mistaken for "infant colic". Rolandic epilepsy involves brief partial and unilateral fits.

240 **TTTFT**

Women with a high risk of having a child with a neural tube defect (first degree relative or personal history, taking anticonvulsants) need 5mg folic acid daily.

241 **TTFTT**

Erythema toxicum is a harmless self limiting skin lesion.

242 **FTFFT**

Decreased skin turgor is 10% dehydration. Sunken fontanelle is seen by 10% dehydration. Drowsiness is at >10% dehydration.

243 **TTTFF**

Gastric lavage and emesis are contraindicated with ingestion of corrosives.

244 **TFFTF**

Stems b and c refer to paracetamol poisoning. With salicylates, drug levels are unreliable until 6 hours after ingestion.

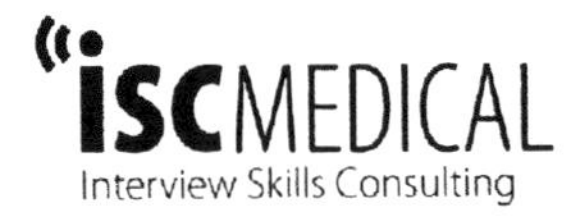

245 **TFFFT**
Papilloedema is a late sign.

246 **FTFTT**
Specific nerve lesions are not infrequently seen.

247 **TFFFF**
Brudzinski's sign is hips flexing on bringing head forward. Lumbar puncture is contraindicated if purpura present. Rashes with meningococcus need not always blanch.

248 **TFTTT**
A continuous or fixed split is a hallmark of ASD.

249 **FTTTF**
They are always generalised. The presence of an infection of the central nervous system is an exclusion criterion.

250 **TTFFF**
Object transfer and weight bearing is expected by 6 months.

251 **FFFFF**
Lorazepam is first choice in status epilepticus. Lamotrigine is useful for absences and Vigabatrin is good for infantile spasms. Carbamazepine may actually exacerbate absence seizures. Ethosuximide, sodium valproate and lamotrigine are useful treatments for absences.

252 **TFTTF**

253 **TTTTT**

254 **TTFTT**

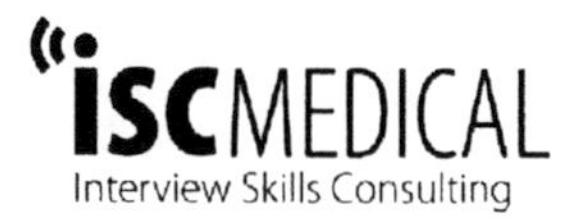

255 **FFTFT**

Testicular feminisation is peripheral androgen insensitivity so male characteristics don't develop. Salt wasting is a feature of CAH where the enzyme defect causes a switch in adrenal biosynthetic pathways with a resultant lack of mineralocorticoids and excess of androgens thereby virulising females. The prepuce should be preserved in hypospadias since it can be used in later repair.

256 **FFTTF**

Listeria = neonate. N. meningitidis = any age. H. Influenzae < 4years.

257 **FFTTT**

Rash begins on the trunk.

258 **FTFFT**

Parvovirus B19 gives a false positive Monospot ® test and is known as slapped cheek virus. It also causes aplastic crises in sickle cell patients.

259 **FFTTF**

Patients are infective for 9 days after the start of parotid swelling.

260 **TFFTF**

Rash starts by the ear then spreads. Patients are infective right from the start of the prodrome. Antibiotics have not be shown to be central to treatment of an identified case.

261 **TFFFT**

PDA, ASD, VSD and AVSD are common.

262 **TFFTT**

Stem b and c are seen later on in life.

263 **TFTTF**

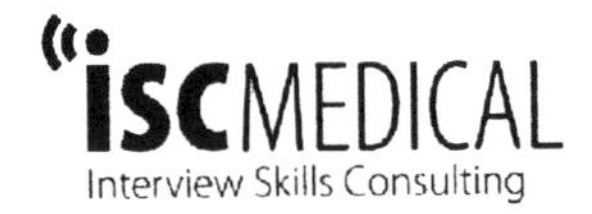

264 **FTFTT**

Aneuploidy is having the incorrect number of chromosomes. Mosaicism is when the genetic makeup of a line of multipotential cells changes from the rest early on in the embryo development. This leads to an embryo having more than the usual one type of genetically unique cell lines.

265 **TTFTT**

Hypotonia is much less common than hypertonia but can be seen with damage to the cerebellum.

266 **TFFFF**

Steroids (prednisolone >2mg/day for > 1 week) within 3 months, or another live vaccine within 3 weeks of considered vaccination, are contraindications to such vaccines being given. HIV is not a contraindication unless there is a severe immunosuppression. Patients with egg allergy can be offered immunisation in hospital in case of anaphylaxis but this is very rare.

267 **FTTFT**

Balloon valvuloplasty is an option for pulmonary stenosis.

268 **FFFTT**

Pica occurs at some stage in most children.

269 **TTTTT**

270 **FFTFT**

There is an equal sex prevalence.

271 **FTFFT**

Iron deficiency anaemia occurs in over 10% of Caucasian. Thalassaemia does cause a microcytic anaemia, but this is not iron deficient. Sodium federate or ferrous fumarate syrup are used most commonly.

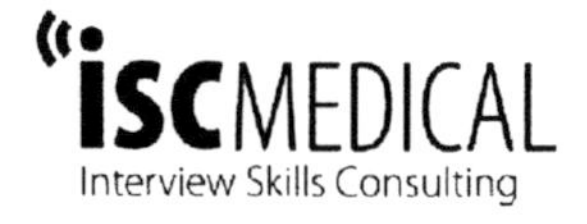

272 **FFTTF**
Infusions should be given when infection is absent.

273 **TTTTF**

274 **FTTFT**
Onset is before 8 years in girls and 9 years in boys.

275 **TFFFF**

276 **TTTTF**

277 **TFFFF**
ASD gives a widely fixed split second heart sound and midsystolic murmur. VSD gives a harsh pansystolic murmur and thrill. Rib notching is a feature of coartation of the aorta. Shock in coarctation is rarely from birth, it is usually a few days later, once after closure of the ductus arteriosus.

278 **FFTFF**
Diphtheria, tetanus, pertussis, Hib MC and polio at 2, 3 and 4 months. MMR at 12-18 months and 4-5yrs. Diphtheria, tetanus, and polio boosters are given at 4-5 yrs and 15-18 yrs. A pertussis booster is given at 4-5 years. Men C is given at 15-24 years if not previously given.

279 **FTTTF**
Projectile vomiting refers to the vomit being projected some distance and suggests pyloric stenosis, whilst effortless regurgitation is normal in many. Vomiting is extremely common and should not be over-investigated unless there are unusual features, poor weight gain or other concerns.

280 **TTTTT**

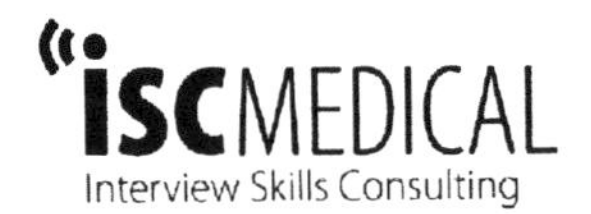

281 **TFFFT**
Ultrasound scanning is specific for scarring following reflux nephropathy but not sensitive enough to exclude it. Ultrasound is best for detecting renal tract anomalies but a DMSA scan should be performed several months after an infection to exclude renal scars.

282 **TFFTF**
Bloody diarrhoea is rarely due to inflammatory bowel disease. Toddler diarrhoea is due to intestinal hurry and resolves by age 4. Liquid stools in an infant is common.

283 **FFTTT**
Kwashiorkor is protein deficiency, Marasmus is caloric deficiency. Parenteral feeding with rehydration can avert renal impairment. Rapid changes electrolyte balances can be dangerous.

284 **TFTFT**
Lead poisoning can cause slow growth.

285 **FFFTT**

286 **TFTTT**

287 **TFTFT**

288 **TFTFT**
Maternal alcohol and short stature are risk factors for IUGR but not prematurity.

289 **FFTTF**
Crying can just mean that a baby isn't getting what it wants.

290 **FTTFF**
There are shared risk factors for prematurity and IUGR such as smoking and infections, but the majority of preterm infants do NOT have IUGR, although slow weight gain after birth is often seen.

291 **TFFFF**

Low birth weight is any baby < 2500g. Preterm is delivery before 37 weeks gestation. Appropriate weight for gestational age can be assessed by comparison to growth tables.

292 **FTTTF**

293 **TTTFT**

294 **TFTFF**

295 **TFTTF**

296 **TFFTT**

A significant proportion of cases have elements of abuse, neglect or medical causes. Coeliacs are intolerant of gluten which is only encountered in food once a baby has been weaned.

297 **FTTTT**

Although attention deficit is noted, hyperactivity is less common than in true attention deficit hyperactivity disorder (ADHD).

298 **FTTFF**

Stem a is Personal-social, stem d is Language and stem e is Personal-social. The purpose of this question and of question 300 is for you to gain an understanding of this type of assessment in term of what skill appears in what category and the order in which skills are attained. We do not suggest that you learn the scale in fine detail. Different adaptations of the Denver scale may contradict one another; our question is based on the scale reproduced in the Oxford handbook of clinical specialties (OUP - 6th edition).

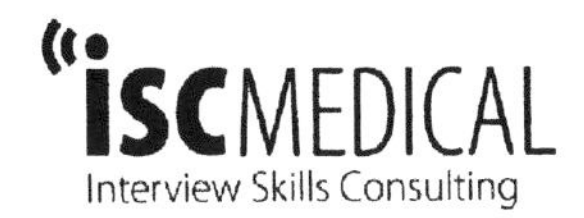

299 **TFTTF**

The definition of SIDS is that after all investigations including autopsy, the death is unexplained. Only theory and speculation guide public health advice. Overheating is a theory and hence using light bedclothes and minimal heating, as well as placing a baby on its back to aid heat loss, is advocated.

300 **TTFFT**

See comment for question 298.

301 **TTFTF**

302 **FTTTF**

Fever is present and often very high.

303 **FFFTT**

This is secondary to respiratory syncytial virus.

304 **TTTTT**

Palatal movement may be paralysed leading to dysarthria.

305 **TTFTF**

Stridor is occasional and often exacerbated by distress to the child.

306 **TFTFT**

It is diphtheria not pertusis which is treated with an antitoxin. Incubation period is 10-14 days.

307 **TFFFF**

There is an excess of cases amongst winter births.

308 **TTTTT**

309 **TFFFF**
The efficacy and safety of St John's Wort has not been fully evaluated, and if patients choose to take it, they must be aware that it can have adverse interaction with other medications.

310 **TTTFF**

311 **FTTTF**

312 **TTTTT**

313 **FTFFF**
Auditory hallucinations may be experienced without mental disorder, e.g. in the context of bereavement, physical illness or exhaustion. A pseudohallucination is where the patient knows that the stimulus, e.g. the voice, is coming from their own mind rather than from elsewhere. Stem d describes a misperception. A delusional perception is when a stimulus triggers a delusional construct e.g. seeing a rainbow means that he has been given a mission to warn everyone that the end of the world is coming. An obsessional thought is persistent, intrusive and often unpleasant but not a hallucination.

314 **FTTTT**

315 **TTTFT**

316 **FFTFT**

317 **FFTTT**
Delirium is an acute organic clouding of consciousness.

318 **TFTTF**

319 **TTTFF**

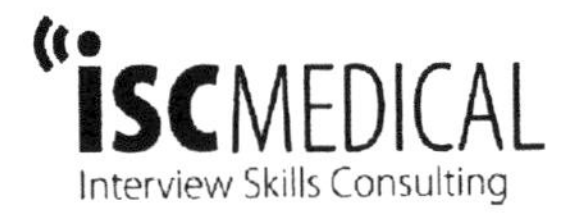

320 **FFTFT**
Edge of seat implies anxiety. Poor eye contact is common to depression. Wild gesticulations often accompany mania.

321 **FTTFT**
Irregular palpitations rather than regular ones suggest a dysrhythmia.

322 **FFFFF**
Hypomania includes all the features of mania but is just a 'watered down' presentation. Stem c defines rapid cycling. Cyclothymia describes a subject who is prone to cyclical mood swings without extreme features of bipolar disorder. Stem d refers to 'Switching'.

323 **TTFFF**

324 **FFFTT**
Lithium is a cause of Type I renal tubular acidosis and of nephrogenic diabetes insipidus.

325 **TFFTT**

326 **TTTFT**
Stem 4 is a test of IQ which isn't formally part of the mental state examination.

327 **TFFTT**

328 **FFFFF**
Stem a describes phobic disorders. Panic disorder tends not to occur with situational cues. Stem d describes social phobia. Agoraphobia often involves fear of crowds of people in which there is no escape. In a panic attack the subject wants it to end, but running away is not thought to be a desire. An intense fear of doom, lack of control and possible impending death is perceived.

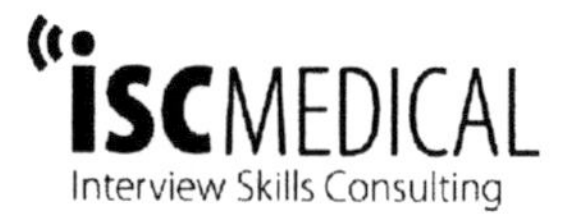

329 TTTFT

Confabulation is seen in Korsakoff's psychosis, to which many patients with Wernicke's will progress, particularly if not given early treatment.

330 FTTFT

Stems a and d are part of the CAGE screening tool which also includes: thoughts to **C**ut down and "**E**ye opener" (a drink taken first thing in the morning). The rest of the dependence syndrome includes: stereotyped drinking, predominance of drink seeking behaviours, drinking to relieve withdrawal symptoms and a failure to maintain abstinence from drinking.

331 FTFTT

332 FTTFT

333 TTFFT

334 TTFTT

335 TTFTF

Cognitive behavioural therapy is a cornerstone of treatment for OCD.

336 TFTFT

Counselling involves listening, reflecting and redefining, but never involves giving advice. Supportive therapy is a combination of counselling, reassurance, encouragement along with other practical assistance e.g. social support to the patient.

337 TTFFT

Melatonin is produced from the pineal gland and there is no firm evidence at present to suggest which wavelength of light performs the best.

338 **TFTTT**

339 **FFTTT**
Steatorrhoea may be seen, but it is usually due to the laxative misuse rather than a feature of the disease itself.

340 **FFTFT**

341 **TFFTT**

342 **TTFTF**
Cigarette smoking lowers their drug levels.

343 **TFFFT**

344 **FFTFT**

345 **FFFFT**
Tricyclics are dangerous in overdose and so best avoided in cases of high suicide risk. Tricyclics are effective in the elderly, however doses may need to be reduced. Tricyclics are less effective than SSRIs, rather than intolerable in children.

346 **TTFFF**

347 **FFTTF**
Side effects can present with a few days of the first dose. Many patients will require several months' continuation of drugs after mood has stabilised. Stopping drugs may also involve a reducing or weaning regimen.

348 **FTFFT**

349 **FTTTF**
ECT is very rarely used in OCD.

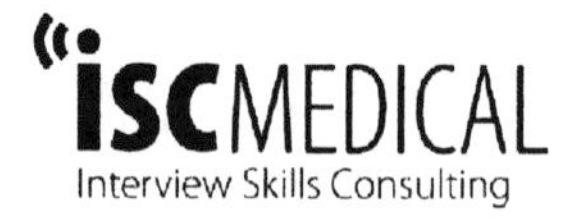

350 **TFFTT**
It is advisable for potential patients not to see others undergoing the procedure.

351 **FTFTT**

352 **FTTFF**
Dysmorphophobia is the concern that one is already deformed or ugly. Stem d is the definition of dissociative disorder and stem e is the definition of somatisation. Of note, somatisation and hypochondriasis are two subtypes of somatoform disorders.

353 **FFFTF**
Stem a describes the 'anxious or avoidant type'. Borderline is also termed emotionally unstable as is described in stem c. Narcissistic is someone who holds a very high opinion of themselves with a feeling of superiority over others. Anankastic is a tendency towards obsessive compulsive behaviour, attention to detail, inflexible and humourless. Stem e describes the 'paranoid' subtype. Schizoid type is humourless, emotionally detached and socially withdrawn.

354 **FFFFT**
In section 2, only one doctor has to be approved as long as the other doctor knows the patient in a professional capacity. The mental health act only applies to treatment when that treatment is directly for the mental disorder and not, as in this case, medical such as heparin. If a patient were to fall unconscious without a prior living will or advanced directive written at a time of lucidity, then emergency treatment can be given under common law. Section 5(2) does not apply to A&E or outpatients. Section 5(4) is only valid up to 6 hours.

355 **TTTFT**

356 **FTFTT**

357 **TTFTT**

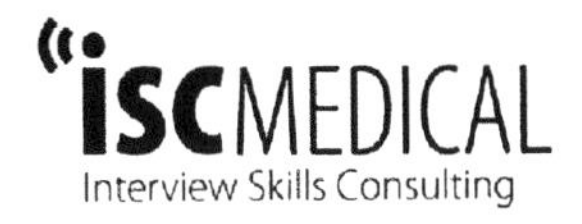

358 **FFTFF**
Avoidance is the problem that must be overcome with anxiety disorders. Systematic desensitisation is a form of gradual exposure to a phobic stimulus which is used in behavioural therapy to overcome the phobia. Flooding is another technique from behavioural therapy where a subject is exposed 'in the deep end' to a phobic stimulus.

359 **FTFFF**
A large trial in 2002 showed no benefit for ginkgo biloba.

360 **TTFTT**

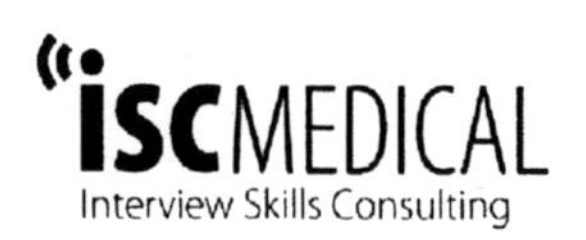
iscMEDICAL
Interview Skills Consulting